World Trade Center Pulmonary Diseases and Multi-Organ System Manifestations

Anthony M. Szema

Editor

World Trade Center Pulmonary Diseases and Multi-Organ System Manifestations

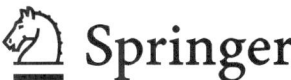 Springer

Editor
Anthony M. Szema
Columbia University Child and Adolescent
  Psychiatric Epidemiology Group
CDC NIOSH U01 0H011308 "9/11 Trauma
  and Toxicity in Childhood: Longitudinal
  Health and Behavioral Outcomes"
New York, NY
USA

Hofstra Northwell School of Medicine at
  Hofstra University
Hempstead, NY
USA

Department of Medicine, Division
  of Pulmonary and Critical Care
Northwell Health
Manhasset, NY
USA

Department of Medicine, Division of
  Allergy/Immunology
Northwell Health
Manhasset, NY
USA

Department of Occupational Medicine,
  Epidemiology, and Prevention
Northwell Health
Manhasset, NY
USA

Stony Brook University Department of
  Technology and Society
College of Engineering and Applied
  Sciences
Stony Brook, NY
USA

RDS2 Solutions
Stony Brook, NY
USA

Three Village Allergy & Asthma, PLLC
Stony Brook, NY
USA

ISBN 978-3-319-59371-5   ISBN 978-3-319-59372-2   (eBook)
DOI 10.1007/978-3-319-59372-2

Library of Congress Control Number: 2017951648

Printed on acid-free paper

This Springer imprint is published by Springer Nature
The registered company is Springer International Publishing AG
The registered company address is: Gewerbestrasse 11, 6330 Cham, Switzerland

Foreword

The terrorist attacks of September 11, 2001, occurring at the World Trade Center in New York City; at the Pentagon in Arlington, Virginia; and in a field near Shanksville, Pennsylvania, led to profound changes in American society. Changes in the security of air travel, expansion of the role of government in homeland security, and an increase in civil society anti-terrorism protections are the most apparent changes to most people. But to those brave women and men who responded to the 9/11 terrorist attacks from all over the USA, and from several foreign countries, and to those survivors (adults and children) who lived nearby the sites which were attacked, they have personally experienced another, more personally troubling change—a decline in their own health.

Since September 11, 2001, a group of healthcare professionals—physicians, nurses, psychologists, and social workers—have provided care for responders and survivors whose health was affected by 9/11. While providing care, these healthcare providers worked hard to understand the medical basis for the signs and symptoms they were seeing in responders and survivors. A significant body of medical science has been generated by these selfless healers in leading scientific publications. Many of these healthcare providers have now authored chapters on the most pervasive physical and mental health conditions seen in 9/11 responders and survivors in a new medical textbook.

As 9/11 medical science grows, more will become known about the long-term effects of the September 11, 2001, attacks on the health of responders and survivors. For now, though, this textbook represents a pioneering effort to bring knowledge about 9/11 health effects to a wider audience of healthcare providers. As more and more 9/11 responders and survivors are now living in every part of the USA, they are likely to present to a healthcare provider who will be grateful for the knowledge contained in this valuable textbook.

John Howard, MD
Administrator, World Trade Center Health Program,
Washington, DC, USA

Acknowledgment

I thank Margaret Moore, Editor, Clinical Medicine, Springer, for the opportunity to edit and contribute to the first edition of the *Textbook of World Trade Center Pulmonary Diseases and Associated Multi-Organ System Manifestations*. Rahul Kumar Sharma, Project Coordinator (Books), and his Springer Nature staff also deserve kudos for making the editing process smooth.

All of our authors are pioneers in the field studying the health consequences of World Trade Center exposure, so this book not only provides the latest scientific and clinical advances but also establishes a historical blueprint for future academicians to study.

Finally, I thank the National Institute for Occupational Safety and Health (NIOSH) director Dr. John Howard for his foreword and support of this project from its incipient stages.

Contents

About the Author

Anthony M. Szema, a member of the Columbia University Child and Adolescent Psychiatric Epidemiology Group, studies lung and immune function among children exposed to the World Trade Center disaster. Szema coined the term World Trade Center Mind Body Lung Injury which describes the dual injury of toxicity and trauma from 9/11. He and colleagues are also beginning a birth cohort epigenetics study among children born on 9/11 in Lower Manhattan. His Editor's Choice paper published in the *JACI* was the first to describe extremely high rates of new-onset asthma in New York City's Chinatown after September 11, 2001. Szema's related work focuses on Iraq and Afghanistan War Lung Injury which is an analogous toxic multifactorial inhalational exposure. Dr. Szema has coinvented a medication which attenuates dust-induced lung injury in animal models and has a seed start-up company which won the Startupalooza in New York City in 2016.

Contributors

Lawrence Amsel Clinical Psychiatry, College of Physicians and Surgeons, Columbia University, New York, NY, USA

New York State Psychiatric Institute, New York, NY, USA

New York Presbyterian Hospital, New York, NY, USA

Evelyn J. Bromet Department of Psychiatry, Stony Brook University, Stony Brook, NY, USA

Caralee Caplan-Shaw Division of Pulmonary and Critical Care Medicine, Department of Medicine, Bellevue Hospital Center/NYU School of Medicine, New York, NY, USA

Alpa G. Desai Division of Pulmonary, Critical Care and Sleep Medicine, HSC 17-040, Stony Brook University, Stony Brook, NY, USA

Talya Greene Department of Community Mental Health, University of Haifa, Haifa, Israel

Raz Gross Division of Psychiatry, The Chaim Sheba Medical Center, Tel Hashomer, Israel

Department of Epidemiology and Preventive Medicine, Sackler Faculty of Medicine, Tel Aviv University, Tel Aviv, Israel

Christina W. Hoven Epidemiology and Psychiatry, Columbia University-NYSPI, New York, NY, USA

Department of Child Psychiatric Epidemiology, Columbia University-NYSPI, New York, NY, USA

Marc Kostrubiak University of Vermont College of Medicine, Burlington, VT, USA

Roman Kotov Department of Psychiatry, Stony Brook University, Stony Brook, NY, USA

Benjamin J. Luft Department of Medicine, Stony Brook University, Stony
Brook, NY, USA

Jacqueline Moline Occupational Medicine, Epidemiology and Prevention,
Hofstra Northwell School of Medicine, Northwell Health, New York, NY, USA

David J. Prezant Fire Department of the City of New York, Bureau of Health
Services, Brooklyn, NY, USA

Joan Reibman Division of Pulmonary and Critical Care Medicine, Department
of Medicine, Bellevue Hospital Center/NYU School of Medicine, New York,
NY, USA

Theresa Schwartz Fire Department of the City of New York, Bureau of Health
Services, Brooklyn, NY, USA

Ankura Singh Fire Department of the City of New York, Bureau of Health
Services, Brooklyn, NY, USA

Gwen S. Skloot Division of Pulmonary, Critical Care and Sleep Medicine, Icahn
School of Medicine at Mount Sinai, New York, NY, USA

Francine R. Smith Northwell Health, New York, NY, USA

Jaime Szeinuk Occupational and Environmental Medicine of Long Island, New
Hyde Park, NY, USA

Department of Occupational Medicine, Epidemiology and Prevention, Hofstra
Northwell School of Medicine, Hempstead, NY, USA

Anthony M. Szema Columbia University Child and Adolescent Psychiatric
Epidemiology Group, CDC NIOSH U01 0H011308 "9/11 Trauma and Toxicity in
Childhood: Longitudinal Health and Behavioral Outcomes", New York, NY, USA

Hofstra Northwell School of Medicine at Hofstra University,
Hempstead, NY, USA

Department of Medicine, Division of Pulmonary and Critical Care,
Northwell Health, Manhasset, NY, USA

Department of Medicine, Division of Allergy/Immunology, Northwell Health,
Manhasset, NY, USA

Department of Occupational Medicine, Epidemiology, and Prevention, Northwell
Health, Manhasset, NY, USA

Stony Brook University Department of Technology and Society,
College of Engineering and Applied Sciences, Stony Brook, NY, USA

RDS2 Solutions, Stony Brook, NY, USA

Three Village Allergy & Asthma, PLLC, Stony Brook, NY, USA

Madeline Vossbrinck Fire Department of the City of New York, Bureau of Health Services, Brooklyn, NY, USA

Elizabeth Ward Intramural Research, American Cancer Society, Atlanta, GA, USA

Mayris P. Webber Department of Epidemiology and Population Health, Montefiore Medical Center and Albert Einstein College of Medicine, Bronx, NY, USA

Fire Department of the City of New York, Bureau of Health Services, Brooklyn, NY, USA

Leigh Wilson Occupational Medicine, Epidemiology and Prevention, Hofstra Northwell School of Medicine, Northwell Health, New York, NY, USA,

Jennifer Yip Fire Department of the City of New York, Bureau of Health Services, Brooklyn, NY, USA

Rachel Zeig-Owens Fire Department of the City of New York, Bureau of Health Services, Brooklyn, NY, USA

The Influence of the WTC Programs on Research

Jacqueline Moline, Leigh Wilson, and Francine R. Smith

Introduction

The attack on the World Trade Center (WTC) buildings on September 11, 2001, resulted in the destruction of the towers and production of a dust plume which exposed workers and residents of Lower Manhattan to a vast array of chemical and physical agents as well as mental and emotional traumatogens. There were fires ignited at the site as the result of 91,000 L of jet fuel from the two airplanes that crashed into the towers in addition to an estimated 490,000 L of transformer oil, 380,000 L of diesel and heating oil, 100,000 tons of organic debris, and fuel from the thousands of cars in the parking structure under the WTC [1]; these burned for 3 months.

The components of the dust plume included particulate matter and products of combustion including but not limited to asbestos, pulverized concrete, glass fibers, crystalline silica, polycyclic aromatic hydrocarbons, polychlorinated biphenyls, furans, organochlorine pesticides, and dioxins as well as combustion products of jet fuel, soot, metals, and volatile organic compounds [2, 3]. The air pollution constituents of the dust plume initially were from both the structural collapse and combustion, though predominantly structural. The cement, ceiling tiles, and drywall contained calcium carbonate, gypsum, vitreous fibers, and calcium sulfate. Windows from the towers contained glass fibers and silicates. Additional materials from the collapse include mercury, benzene, volatile organic compounds (VOCs), chlorodifluoromethane, heavy metals, hydrogen sulfide, and inorganic acids. The dust plume also affected indoor air quality, infiltrating homes and offices, with up to several

J. Moline (✉) • L. Wilson
Occupational Medicine, Epidemiology and Prevention, Hofstra Northwell
School of Medicine, Northwell Health, Great Neck, NY 11021, USA
e-mail: jmoline@northwell.edu; lwilson8@northwell.edu

F.R. Smith
Northwell Health, New York, NY 11042, USA
e-mail: FSmith1@northwell.edu

© Springer International Publishing AG 2018
A.M. Szema (ed.), *World Trade Center Pulmonary Diseases and Multi-Organ System Manifestations*, DOI 10.1007/978-3-319-59372-2_1

inches in some cases [4]. Asbestos was used as insulation and a fire retardant in the World Trade Center towers. The composition of the dust evolved as rescue and recovery began, with organic hydrocarbons, polynuclear aromatic hydrocarbons (PAHs), and diesel exhaust from fires, combustion, and engines becoming the main airborne exposures [5]. Health consequences from these airborne exposures include airway irritation and cancer [2, 3, 6–10]. The makeup of the dust plume likely evolved rapidly once initiated; unfortunately, this remains uncertain, since there were no air samples available from September 11, 2001, as there were no air sampling devices operating in close proximity to the WTC site. In the days following the collapse of the buildings, environmental researchers and a number of state and federal agencies collected settled dust. Ambient air samples were first collected on September 18, 2001, in an effort to characterize human exposure. There were hundreds of thousands of samples of outdoor air, bulk dust, and indoor air and wipe samples in addition to personal air samples from worker breathing zones [11].

Concerns regarding the toxins created by this disaster and possible health effects of exposure to the WTC disaster site were recognized early on by the New York City Department of Health and Mental Hygiene (NYCDOHMH) [5]. The NYCDOHMH reached out to the CDC to conduct occupational health exposure assessments for the firefighters and emergency medical technicians at the WTC disaster site. The National Institute of Environmental Health Sciences Superfund Basic Science Research Program conveyed a meeting in New Jersey in late September 2001 to discuss possible research projects. This meeting led to some of the earliest research funding related to the WTC disaster.

As a result of this partnership with the CDC, the Fire Department of the City of New York (FDNY) began a medical monitoring program within 1 month of September 11 to evaluate the health of the FDNY members who were at the site. Comparisons of firefighters exposed on 9/11 and those without exposure were also performed, providing additional information [12].

Adverse health effects in workers and volunteers at the WTC cleanup site and Staten Island landfill were initially reported in descriptive articles reporting a high frequency of upper and lower respiratory signs and symptoms including persistent cough, wheeze, shortness of breath, new diagnoses of asthma, reactive airways dysfunction syndrome/irritant-induced asthma, sinusitis, and laryngitis [13–15]. Case reports describing exposed individuals with persistent respiratory symptoms led to investigations such as bronchoscopies, and lung biopsies revealing diagnoses including but not limited to acute eosinophilic pneumonia, granulomatous pneumonitis, and bronchiolitis obliterans [16–18].

History of the WTC Health Program

Due to concerns for the health of workers participating in the rescue and recovery effort at the WTC disaster site, the WTC Worker and Volunteer Medical Screening Program began July 16, 2002. This program was similar in scope to the newly established FDNY Program for Core Clinical Evaluation and Medical Monitoring Services [19]. Funded by the National Institute for Occupational Safety and Health (NIOSH) and the Centers for Disease Control and Prevention (CDC), this multicenter consortium was established to provide a free standardized physical and mental health screening program to non-FDNY WTC responders involved in rescue, recovery, restoration of services, and cleanup. In 2003, Congress appropriated $90 million to implement longer-term monitoring for the WTC responders. Rather than awarding contracts solely to FDNY and Mount Sinai School of Medicine (MSSM), separate contracts were awarded to participating occupational medicine centers. In addition to FDNY, contracts were given to MSSM, Bellevue Occupational Health, the State University of New York (SUNY), Stony Brook Occupational Medicine, Queens College—Center for the Biology of Natural Systems, and the University of Medicine and Dentistry of New Jersey—Robert Wood Johnson Medical School. The goal was to continue the provision of care at regional clinical centers with occupational medicine expertise in more convenient locations for the majority of responders.

Treatment for WTC-related health conditions of responders was initially funded through philanthropy, but in November of 2006, federal funds became available for treatment and allowed for expansion of services to this population. From the WTC Workers and Volunteer Screening and Monitoring Program, the World Trade Center Medical Monitoring and Treatment Program (WTC MMTP) was established. A change of the program title also meant a change in funding and covered services for responders. The program evolved to provide annual medical surveillance examinations to assess health status, identify health conditions related to exposures at the WTC site, and deliver comprehensive care for WTC-related medical conditions, including physical and mental health and social work services. Estimates from 50,000 to 90,000 workers are believed to have participated in activities as first responders at the WTC disaster site, with the true number thought to be closer to 60,000–70,000 [20]. Data published in Environmental Health Perspectives [13] from the early years of the program revealed that of the 9,442 responders who presented to the program between July 2002 and April 2004, 69% reported new or worsening respiratory symptoms while performing work at the WTC site; in addition, 59% reported that the symptoms persisted at the time of their exam. Among those reporting respiratory symptoms and were asymptomatic prior to September 11, 2001, 61% reported that their respiratory symptoms began while working on the WTC effort. Twenty-eight percent of these responders had abnormal spirometry (in 21% FVC was low and 5% had evidence of obstruction).

On January 2, 2011, President Obama signed the James Zadroga 9/11 Health and Compensation Act of 2010 (Zadroga Act) into law. This law amended the Public Health Service Act, establishing the WTC Health Program, to be administered by the NIOSH, part of the CDC, within the US Department of Health and Human Services. Instead of requiring the WTC MMTP Consortium clinics to reapply to the CDC for funds annually, a 5-year contract for funding was available for these clinics. The centers that applied for and were awarded these contracts in 2011 are part of what is now called the World Trade Center Health Program [21]. In the Zadroga

Act, three specific cohorts were defined: the FDNY cohort (FDNY and FDNY EMS), the responder cohort (rescue and recover workers), and the survivor cohort (building reoccupants in the downtown area, residents below Canal Street, students and teachers, and those exposed on 9/11/01). The Zadroga Act was reauthorized in 2016 for 75 additional years providing resources to pay for medical conditions related to the World Trade Center as well as research funding.

Pulmonary Findings

Early research focused on the health effects of the dust and implications for adverse health effects. WTC dust was collected from different locations in Lower Manhattan near the WTC site on September 12 and 13, and additional dust was collected the following week [3, 22, 23]. Multiple chemicals, products of combustion, construction materials, and metals were found. One notable finding in the settled dust was a highly alkaline pH (9.0–11.0) (Fig. 1).

Dust samples were used in toxicological evaluations. Gavett compared WTC dust (PM2.5) to similar-sized PM2.5 dust from Mount Saint Helens' dust, residual of fly ash, and National Institute of Standards and Technology (NIST) standard reference material 1649a (urban PM2.5 dust from Washington DC). Rodents that died at a relatively high level (100 mg) of WTC dust show a mild to moderate degree of pulmonary inflammation, but it was not as severe as the inflammation noted with residual oil fly ash (ROFA) or the NIST 1649a dust. However, rodents exposed to the same dose of WTC PM2.5 dust experienced a significant degree of airway hyperresponsiveness as measured by methacholine aerosol [25].

Work published in the *New England Journal of Medicine* by Prezant et al. in 2002 defined and described "World Trade Center Cough Syndrome" as well as other symptoms present in a sample of FDNY firefighters with varied degrees of exposure at the WTC site. WTC Cough Syndrome was defined as persistent cough that developed following WTC exposure and was sufficiently severe to result in 4 or more weeks of medical leave. Evaluations included spirometry, a standardized questionnaire, chest imaging, and airway responsiveness testing. Results included presence of WTC Cough Syndrome in 8% of 6,958 firefighters in the group identified with the highest level of exposure, 3% of 1,320 with the defined "moderate" level of exposure, and 1% of the 1,320 with low-level exposure. From October 1 to 14, 2001, a methacholine or bronchodilator challenge for bronchial hyperreactivity was performed on 102 firefighters with moderate to high levels of exposure to inorganic dusts, pyrolysis products, etc., on September 11, 2001. None of the firefighters were out on medical leave, and all had reported cough within 24 hours of exposure on September 11, 2001. Twenty-three percent of firefighters with high levels of exposure also had bronchial hyperreactivity [15].

FDNY firefighters in the highest stratified exposure group had 23% hyperreactivity (as defined by methacholine PCO2 ≤8 mg/mL) compared with 11% moderately exposed with hyperreactivity. FDNY rescue workers vs. 11% in the moderately

Sample	Street		
	Cortlandt	Cherry	Market
Color	Pinkish gray	Pinkish gray	Pinkish gray
pH	11.5	9.2	9.3
Nonfiber (cement/carbon: %)[a]	50.0	49.2	37.0
Glass fiber (%)[a]	40.0	40.0	40.0
Cellulose (%)[a]	9.2	10.0	20.0
Chrysotile asbestos (%)[a]	0.8	0.8	3.0
Aerodynamically seperated sample (% mass)			
< 2.5 μm diameter	1.12	0.88	1.30
2.5–10 μm diameter	0.35	0.30	0.40
10–53 μm diameter	37.03	46.61	34.69
> 53 μm diameter	61.50	52.21	63.60
Sieved sample (% mass)			
< 75 μm diameter	38.00	30.00	37.00
75–300 μm diameter	46.0	49.00	42.00
> 300 μm diameter	16.0	23.00	21.0
Anions/cations (ng/g)			
Fluoride	220	70	ND
Chloride	800	270	220
Nitrate	330	ND	ND
Sulfate	41.400	35.200	42.100
Calcium	18.200	14.000	17.700
Sodium	400	200	130
Potassium	60	170	270

ND, not detectable.
[a]Values reported to L.C. Chen by the Ambient Group, TNC (New York, NY), measured by polarized light microscopy (400–450x).

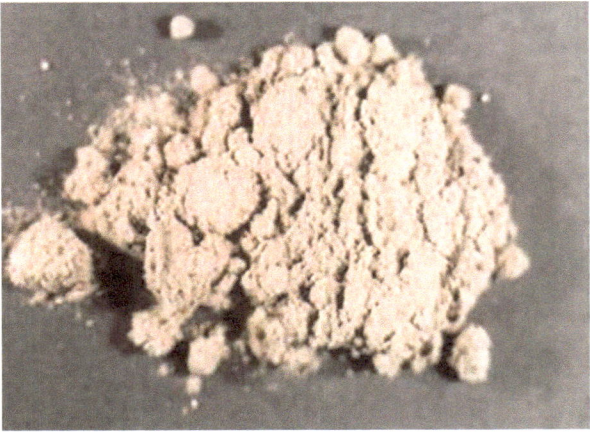

Fig. 1 A table listing characteristics of WTC dust and a figure of the dust that settles near the WTC disaster site [24]

exposed group and 4% reactivity of controls, as defined by nonexposed FDNY members, had evidence of persistent airway hyperreactivity at 1 year; 16% of the highly exposed FDNY workers met criteria for reactive airways dysfunction syndrome. The results from both the animal and human studies showed that exposure to WTC dust caused increased bronchial hyperreactivity.

Later work by Prezant et al. documented evidence of an exposure gradient which cited that 57% of 8,418 WTC registry participants who were caught in the dust cloud reported new or worsening respiratory symptoms after exposure. Over time, World Trade Center Cough Syndrome was further described as a "chronic cough syndrome" which was the consequence of upper and lower respiratory tract disease manifesting as cough. Disorders of the upper airway included reactive upper airways dysfunction syndrome, chronic rhinosinusitis, and gastroesophageal reflux disease in combination or individually. Lower airway causes of chronic cough were often identified with other symptoms such as shortness of breath, chest tightness, and decreased exercise tolerance, and attributed to asthma, reactive airways dysfunction syndrome, and asthma-bronchitis overlap syndrome (in some cases, other etiologies such as sarcoidosis, bronchiolitis, or pulmonary fibrosis were identified) [26].

In September 2011, Wisnivesky et al. published a review of persistent illnesses in rescue workers from the WTC site. Data from 27,449 participants in the "WTC Screening, Monitoring and Treatment Program" (now known as the World Trade Center Health Program) reported the 9-year cumulative incidence rates for the most common WTC-related conditions: asthma 27.6% (representing 7,027 members), sinusitis 42.3% (5,870), and gastroesophageal reflux disease (GERD) 39.3% (5,650). In police officers, depression was 7.0% (3,648 members), post traumatic stress disorder (PTSD) 9.3% (3,761), and panic disorder 8.4% (3,780). In other rescue and recovery workers, cumulative incidence of depression was 27.5% (4200 members), PTSD 31.9% (4,342), and panic disorder 21.2% (4,953). A 9-year cumulative incidence for spirometric abnormalities was 41.8% (5,769 members), with low forced vital capacity making up 75% of these abnormalities. Highest level of exposure was correlated with members having the greatest number of disorders. Physical health conditions were frequently comorbid with mental health disorders [27].

Sarcoidosis and Sarcoid-Like Granulomatous Disease

Work by the responder cohort, FDNY, and the World Trade Center Health Registry evaluated whether there is a higher than expected rate of sarcoidosis and sarcoid-like granulomatous disease among WTC responders and registry enrollees.

Izbicki et al. studied the incidence of biopsy-proven sarcoidosis and sarcoid-like granulomatous pulmonary disease in 26 cases of FDNY rescue workers (23 firefighters, 3 EMS) identified in the 5 years following September 11, 2001. Sarcoidosis is a multisystem noncaseating granulomatous disease typically affecting young to middle-aged adults and predominantly involving the lungs, lymph nodes, and skin, all of which are thought to be potential sites of entry for immunogenic occupational and environmental exposures. Although the etiology of sarcoidosis is not well understood, some infectious and occupational agents have been implicated due to their immunogenicity. All 26 cases had intrathoracic adenopathy, and 18 had findings consistent with concomitant asthma. All cases had pre-hire chest X-rays which were negative for findings suggestive of granulomatous disease and normal spirometry; in addition, every 3 years, these workers had chest X-rays as part of the medical monitoring program. Cases were stratified based on whether they were in evaluation for symptoms (17 cases) or found on monitoring chest X-ray (9 cases). Thirteen of the cases were identified in the year after September 11, 2001 (calculated incidence rate of 86/100,000), and according to the authors' calculations, the overall 5-year relative risk following exposure at Ground Zero was 2.36 (2.36; 95% confidence interval, 1.17–4.78; $p = 0.017$) [28].

Jordan et al. [29] performed case-control analysis of biopsy-proven cases of sarcoidosis diagnosed post-September 11, 2001, among WTC Health Registry enrollees. Controls were matched to cases on age, sex, race/ethnicity, and the case's WTC registry status (responder or survivor). This study included 28 cases and 109 controls and identified "working on the debris pile" as carrying an elevated risk for sarcoidosis; however, dust cloud exposure was not an independent risk factor [29].

Crowley et al. [30] described 38 patients classified as "definite" cases and calculated a 6-year incidence rate of 192/100,000 with the peak incidence of 54 per 100,000 person-years between September 11, 2003, and September 11, 2004. They found nearly double the incidence in black vs white responders. Low FVC was the most common spirometric abnormality.

Other Persistent PFT Abnormalities

In 2009, Skloot et al. published the first longitudinal study of lung function among WTC responders. Skloot et al. found that lung function improved in never smokers with hyperresponsiveness between exams 1 and 2 but not in smokers [31]. Berger described 58 patients with reduced vital capacity, FRC, TLC, and preserved FEV1/FVC who after thorough evaluation have no evidence of parenchymal, chest wall, or neuromuscular disease. The authors propose that the decrease in TLC is the result of functional abnormalities in the distal lung attributable to WTC dust exposure (reduced TLC differentiates this group of subjects from patients with ILD as TLC is not known to be a hallmark of ILD) [32].

A case-control study was conducted which identified 180 people from the World Trade Center Health Registry who reported persistent "lower respiratory symptoms": cough, wheeze, and shortness of breath, compared with 473 control subjects. Nineteen percent of cases vs 11% of controls were found to have abnormal spirometry ($p < 0.05$). In addition, impulse oscillometry which was measuring airway resistance revealed higher airway resistance in cases than controls, suggesting distal airway dysfunction may be a mechanism for symptoms [33].

Banauch et al. measured bronchial hyperresponsiveness in FDNY-exposed firefighters. FDNY researchers evaluated pulmonary function declines among FDNY firefighters and emergency medical service workers stratified by arrival time at the WTC site (as a surrogate for intensity of exposure). In the first year after 9/11, there was an average 372 mL decline in forced expiratory volume in the first second (FEV1) compared to a normal annual decline of 31 mL in the 5 years prior to September 11 [34]. The proportion of nonsmoking firefighters with an FEV1 below the lower limit of normal increased from 3% to 18% for firefighters and from 12% to 22% for EMS workers. Follow-up evaluations after 6 years showed that pulmonary function did not recover to pre-9/11 levels but did not appear to decline beyond normally expected levels [35]. While the predominant spirometric abnormality among FDNY rescue workers was a decreased forced expiratory volume in 1 second (FEV1) [36], persistent spirometric abnormalities, notably decreased forced vital capacity (FVC), were noted among non-FDNY responders [31]. Banauch found that FDNY rescue workers with mild to moderate α1-antitrypsin deficiency had significant decline accelerations in FEV1 above normal aging-related declines [37]. The authors postulated that this represented a mild gene-by-environment interaction. Cough was also persistent in many WTC-exposed firefighters with α1-antitrypsin deficiency.

Pulmonary function tests among New York City Police Department (NYPD) emergency service unit workers showed higher rates of pulmonary function test abnormalities and bronchodilation response in officers with higher-intensity exposure [38]. Skloot found abnormal forced oscillometry indicating large airway dysfunction in WTC-exposed ironworkers who did not wear canister respirators [39]. Oppenheimer studied 174 individuals who had WTC exposure, pulmonary symptoms, and normal spirometry [40]. The authors found elevated airway resistance and frequency dependence of resistance determined by impedance oscillometry, heterogeneity of distal airway function, and reversibility of functional abnormalities to or toward normal following bronchodilator administration. Oppenheimer concluded that dysfunction in airways distal to those evaluated by spirometry might be the reason for the symptoms [40].

Cancer

Due to the numerous known and probable human carcinogens present in the dust at the WTC site, there is biological plausibility for exposure-related cancers to develop in the exposed population. As of October 2012, the World Trade Center Health Program began the process of surveillance and care for many types of cancer. Given the anticipated long and varied latencies for cancer, the data related to cancer surveillance is in its infancy. Data presented in this article describes 20,984 rescue workers and 575 cancers in 552 individuals. For all cancer sites combined, the overall SIR = 1.15 and 95% CI, 1.06 and 1.25 [41].

Moline et al. reported on eight histologically confirmed cases of multiple myeloma (MM) among 28,252 WTC responders for which there was known age and gender data. In their report, exposure to benzene, PAHs, polychlorinated biphenyls, and other organochlorines were cited as possible sources for toxicity that may have contributed to the development of this disease. The authors noted that overall 6.8 cases of MM would have been expected and only 1.2 of those cases in responders under 45; however, four of their cases were under 45 (5.6 would have been expected in the over 45 group and four were documented) [20].

Zeig-Owens et al. published in *The Lancet* an evaluation of cancer incidence in 9,853 men who were employed as firefighters as of January 1, 1996, and were exposed at the WTC site. This cohort was compared with other nonexposed firefighters and with the general population. It was found that 7 years after September 11, 2001, firefighters exposed to WTC dust at a standardized incidence ratio of 1.19 were 19% more likely to have a cancer diagnosis; this was reportedly corrected for surveillance bias [42].

Zadroga Act

The Zadroga Act amends the Public Health Service Act. It ensures the provision of medical monitoring and treatment to "eligible firefighters and related personnel, law enforcement officers, and rescue, recovery and cleanup workers who responded to the September 11, 2001 terrorist attacks in New York City, Shanksville, PA, and the Pentagon, and to eligible survivors of the New York City attacks [43]." The Zadroga Act ensures contracts with Clinical Centers of Excellence and Data Centers. The Clinical Centers of Excellence (CCEs) provide the evaluation, medical monitoring and treatment services, outreach, and translation services to responders. The Data Centers are available "for receiving, analyzing, and reporting to the WTC Program Administrator on data that have been collected and reported by the corresponding Clinical Centers of Excellence." These services are provided at no cost to enrolled WTC responders and survivors [21].

In 2015 the CDC published a draft WTC Health Program Research-to-Care Logic Model and Narrative. This document illustrates and describes the inputs, activities, outputs and short-, intermediate-, and long-term outcomes of members [44] (Fig. 2).

Data Center Mandates

The Zadroga Act also gives a description of what information the Data Center should be collecting and providing. It should be providing a means of uniform data collection across all clinical centers. This includes developing uniform monitoring

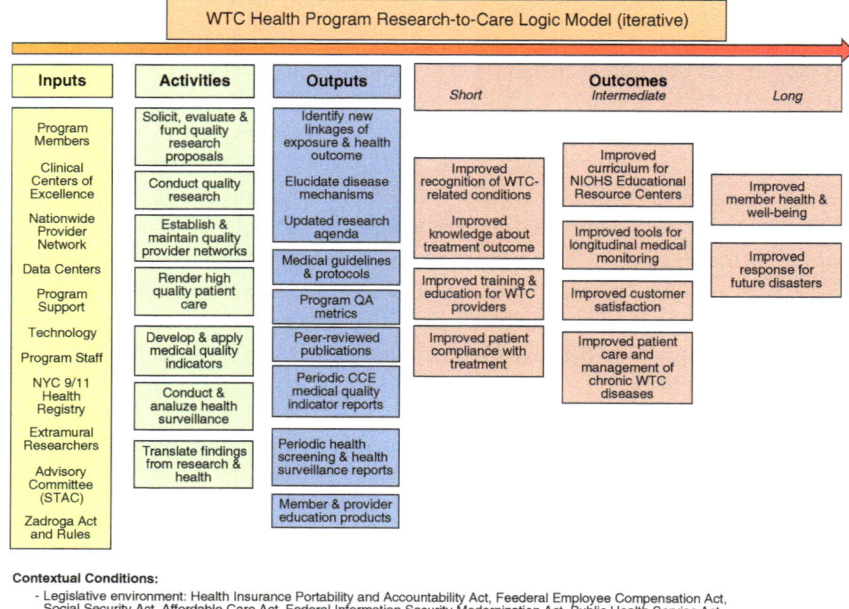

Fig. 2 WTC Health Program Research-to-Care Logic Model [44]

and initial health evaluation and treatment protocols with respect to WTC-related health conditions. The Data Center coordinates outreach activities with the CCEs and the administration of activities with the WTC Health Program Steering Committee. Collaboration between the Data Center and the World Trade Center Health Registry is required.

When research funding became available in 2011, the amount of patients that had been seen for mental health problems, instead of physical health problems, motivated researchers to apply for research funding to investigate further into the subject matter. Additionally, early papers investigating exposure and cancer in WTC responders [20, 45–48] led to an additional request for proposal (RFP) in 2012, allotting for coverage and additional dollars for treatment of WTC-related cancers.

As part of the Zadroga Act, funding for research related to the aftermath of the WTC became available in 2011. The number of grants awarded has steadily increased since 2011. As of 2016 with the reauthorization of the Zadroga Act, a yearly RFP for research projects occurs.

Since 2011 a total of 53 research projects have been funded. Table 1 lists the titles and year of the funded research.

Table 1 WTC research grants funded 2011–2016 [49]

Year	Title
2011	Burden of mental-physical comorbidity in World Trade Center responders
2011	Cancer among WTC responders: enhanced surveillance, exposure assessment, and cancer specific risks
2011	Cardiovascular health impact
2012	Biomarkers of psychological risk and resilience in World Trade Center responders
2012	Bronchial reactivity and the course of lung function
2012	Epigenetic linkage between PTSD and respiratory disease in WTC responders
2012	Extension of the World Trade Center Health Registry
2012	For how long is WTC exposure associated with incident airway obstruction?
2012	Obstructive sleep apnea in WTC responders: role of nasal pathology
2012	Prognosis and determinants of asthma morbidity in WTC rescue and recovery workers
2012	Pulmonary diseases in WTC workers: symptoms, function, and chest CT correlates
2012	Service need and use among youth exposed to the WTC attack
2012	The impact of 9/11 on youth: mental health, substance use, and other risk behaviors
2013	Early identification of World Trade Center conditions in adolescents
2013	Mind body treatment for WTC responders with comorbid PTSD and respiratory illness
2013	Post-9/11 incidence of systemic autoimmune diseases in the FDNY cohort
2013	Prostate cancer risk and outcome of WTC respondents
2013	Trace elements in autopsy tissues from World Trade Center decedents
2013	Uncontrolled lower respiratory symptoms in the WTC survivor program
2014	Assessing the impacts of epidemiologic biases in WTC health studies
2014	Biorepository of cancer tissue samples from WTC responders
2014	Deciphering biological linkages between PTSD and respiratory disease in WTC responders
2014	Evolution of risk factors for sinusitis in WTC exposed firefighters
2014	For how long is WTC exposure associated with chronic rhinosinusitis?
2014	Mental health impact and service use among Asian survivors and rescuers exposed to the WTC attack
2014	Post-9/11 cancer incidence in FDNY firefighters
2014	Renal and cardiovascular impairment in WTC responders: implications for diagnosis and treatment
2014	The daily burden of PTSD and respiratory problems in World Trade Center responders
2014	WTC-heart: a cohort study of heart disease in World Trade Center responders
2015	A pilot test of the relaxation response resiliency program (3RP) in Spanish-speaking World Trade Center disaster survivors with PTSD
2015	Childhood exposures to persistent organic pollutants in the World Trade Center disaster and cardiovascular consequences
2015	Child characteristics and outcomes of WTC-associated sarcoidosis

(continued)

Table 1 (continued)

Year	Title
2015	Cognitive function among World Trade Center rescue and recovery workers—direct mediation through comorbidities
2015	Context and ethnic diversity: children's responses to 9/11
2015	Enhanced assessment of WTC exposure and global DNA methylation
2015	Gene expression profiles as markers of PTSD risk and resilience in WTC responders
2016	Extension of the World Trade Center Health Registry
2016	Head and neck cancer in the World Trade Center health program cohort; elucidating risk factors to reduce incidence and morbidity
2016	Evolution of risk factors for lung function decline in WTC exposed firefighters
2016	Maintenance and extension of a cohort of career firefighters as non-WTC exposed comparison for the FDNY firefighter cohort
2016	Small airway chronic obstructive disease syndrome following exposure to WTC dust
2016	World Trade Center exposures, neuropathic symptoms and nervous system injury
2016	RDoC domains underlying emotional health and trajectories of psychopathology in families of WTC first responders and evacuees: a genome-wide GxE study
2016	9/11 trauma and toxicity in childhood: longitudinal health and behavioral outcomes
2016	Incidence, latency, and survival of cancer following World Trade Center exposure
2016	Hepatitis C virus infection in WTC responders
2016	Structural and functional neuroimaging of post-traumatic stress disorder and cognitive impairment in World Trade Center responders
2016	Thyroid cancer risk in WTC responders
2016	Assessing inflammatory and behavioral pathways linking PTSD to increased asthma morbidity in WTC workers
2016	Impact of WTC dust on immune functions and prostate cancer promotion
2016	Roles for WTC dust and DEP co-pollutant in first responder cardiovascular ailments
2016	A randomized controlled trial of Internet CBT for PTSD in WTC responders
2016	Personality-informed care model for 9/11-related comorbid conditions

There were 11 pulmonary projects funded as of 2016 which are described in Table 2.

Table 3 lists scholarly journal articles that were published as a result of the funding of the pulmonary research projects in Table 2.

Table 2 WTC pulmonary research grants [49]

2011	Title: Burden of mental–physical comorbidity in World Trade Center responders
	Synopsis of project: The study objective is to test mechanisms thought to be responsible for the comorbidity between psychiatric and medical sequelae of World Trade Center (WTC) exposures. We propose to study responders participating in the WTC Health Programs. Of the entire cohort, approximately 16,000 completed the first two monitoring visits, about 2 years apart. In addition to routine questionnaires completed by responders at their monitoring visits, we conduct standard interviews designed to diagnose WTC-related post-traumatic stress disorder (PTSD). The longitudinal data will allow us to evaluate potential mechanisms underlying the links between mental and physical disorders
2012	Title: Biomarkers of psychological risk and resilience in World Trade Center responders
	Synopsis of project: This study will employ a multilevel approach to study clinical, psychosocial, neuroendocrine, genotypic, gene-environment interaction, and molecular factors associated with PTSD risk and resilience in a sample of 500 WTC responders. The study will provide important information about the risk and resilience factors for PTSD in disaster responders and make possible the development of improved preventive and treatment interventions for this disorder in disaster responders and trauma-exposed individuals in general
2012	Title: Bronchial reactivity and the course of lung function
	Synopsis of project: Persistent obstructive airways disease (an asthma-like condition) is common among World Trade Center-exposed firefighters, though rare in this population before September 11, 2001. In about 30%, there is accompanying bronchial hyperreactivity (easily triggered airway narrowing). This study will reexamine a large number of firefighters who had bronchial reactivity soon after 9/11 to determine whether those with bronchial hyperreactivity at onset have persistent hyperactivity more than 10 years later, whether they have accelerated lung function decline, and whether those treated with anti-asthma medications were more likely to show resolution of bronchial hyperactivity or show less rapid decline in lung function
2012	Title: Epigenetic linkage between PTSD and respiratory disease in WTC responders
	Synopsis of project: World Trade Center disaster responders exhibit persistent symptoms of post-traumatic stress disorder (PTSD) and respiratory illness linked to the severity of their exposures. One-quarter of responders affected by these conditions suffer from both, resulting in increased disability and utilization of medical services. This study will examine the potential mechanisms underlying PTSD/respiratory comorbidity that may facilitate the development of more effective, theory-driven interventions for these difficult to treat patients
2012	Title: For how long is WTC exposure associated with incident airway obstruction?
	Synopsis of project: The study uses innovative statistical methods—parametric survival models with change points—to study the incidence of new-onset obstructive airway disease (OAD) diagnoses and symptoms over the first 10 years following WTC exposure, with the goal of determining the length of time that exposure response gradients are observed among exposed FDNY firefighters. This study will allow estimation of the length of time that a relatively short-term, high-intensity exposure may be associated with incident respiratory illness

(continued)

Table 2 (continued)

2012	Title: Health and socioeconomic sequelae of the WTC disaster among responders
	Synopsis of project: Overall health status of WTC responders was evaluated by comparing prevalence of five major health outcomes to the general population surveyed by the National Health Interview Survey (NHIS). Potential associations between new onset of asthma and WTC exposures were investigated, especially the protective effect of respirator use during rescue and recovery activities. A total of 26,796 responders who participated in the WTC Health Program (WTCHP) from 2002 to 2010 were included in the analysis. Standardized morbidity ratios (SMR) were calculated after adjusting for age and occupation, separately, and stratified by gender. Self-reported lifetime prevalence of each outcome was used for SMR. Internal comparison was conducted for asthma incidence. Incidence rate ratios (IRR) were estimated using the generalized estimating equations with robust Poisson family and log link. SMR for asthma was the only outcome showing an elevated rate compared to the general population. From the internal comparison, protective service (IRR = 1.31 (1.12–1.54)) and utility workers (IRR = 1.39 (1.11–1.73)) had a higher risk of experiencing asthma compared to construction workers. Responders who arrived at the site on 9/11 not in the dust cloud (IRR = 0.81 (0.71–0.93)) or later had a lower risk of getting asthma than those who arrived on 9/11 in the dust cloud. Notably, responders who used a full-/half-face respirator on September 11 to September 18 had a significantly lower risk (IRR = 0.70 (0.60–0.82)) than when none was worn. We confirmed that asthma was the main health problem among WTC responders, though we did not observe an increased risk of the other four health outcomes. We also found a clear protective effect of using a respirator on asthma incidence. This is an important finding not only for future disaster preparedness but also for protecting general workers from their daily occupational exposures
2012	Title: Obstructive sleep apnea in WTC responders: role of nasal pathology
	Synopsis of project: Obstructive sleep apnea (OSA) is a highly prevalent disorder with significant morbidity and impact on quality of life that can be improved by treatment with continuous positive airway pressure (CPAP). This study will examine the role of nasal pathology in World Trade Center (WTC) responders in the development of OSA and its impact on their ability to use CPAP. The present study contributes to understanding the relationship of nasal/upper airway mechanisms to the development of sleep apnea in this population and explores the possibility of improving comfort and adherence to CPAP treatment by modifying how CPAP is delivered
2012	Title: Pulmonary diseases in WTC workers: symptoms, function, and chest CT correlates
	Synopsis of project: The overall goal of this study is to identify the early manifestations of lung disease among the World Trade Center (WTC) workers and volunteers, as well as investigate their risk factors. The study team will perform standardized and computer-assisted readings of all chest CT scans received by WTC workers and volunteers at the Mount Sinai Medical Center since January 2003; assess the findings in a systematic way; evaluate the correlation of findings with clinical, functional, and exposure indicators; and develop a protocol for continued radiological surveillance of this cohort
2013	Title: Uncontrolled lower respiratory symptoms in the WTC survivor program
	Synopsis of project: Many "survivors" (community members) in the World Trade Center (WTC) clinical treatment program have persistent lower respiratory symptoms (LRS) despite treatment. This study will test the hypothesis that patients with uncontrolled LRS have (despite aggressive medical therapy) increased rates of abnormal airway physiology, airway inflammation, and comorbid conditions when compared to those with controlled symptoms. Identifying these mechanisms for uncontrolled LRS is imperative to guide therapy with the important potential to reduce secondary adverse health outcomes

Table 2 (continued)

2014	Title: Deciphering biological linkages between PTSD and respiratory disease in WTC responders
	Synopsis of project: The September 11, 2001, terrorist attack on the World Trade Center was an extraordinary environmental disaster resulting in an unprecedented combination of physical and emotional trauma. As many as 60% of responders will experience clinically significant symptoms, most prominently post-traumatic stress disorder (PTSD) and lower respiratory symptoms (LRS). Our group found that PTSD is not only associated with LRS but may contribute to the development of these symptoms as well as diminish their response to treatment. We have performed epigenetic studies and are beginning to untangle the genes responsible for this association. The proposed study will extend these findings to identify the precise cell where these pathogenic relationships are occurring. Ultimately, this knowledge will lead to the development of better diagnostics and more specific treatment for this disease process
2014	Title: The daily burden of PTSD and respiratory problems in World Trade Center responders
	Synopsis of project: Comorbid post-traumatic stress disorder (PTSD) and lower respiratory symptoms (LRS) are among the most common and persistent health burdens faced by World Trade Center (WTC) responders following the attacks on 9/11. For the first time, the proposed study will use ecological momentary assessment approach to survey WTC responders in real time about the prevalence, burden, and the sequence of PTSD and LRS and to test biological processes involved

Table 3 Papers published from WTC pulmonary research grants [49]

Longitudinal study of the impact of psychological distress symptoms on new-onset upper gastrointestinal symptoms in World Trade Center responders, Psychosomatic Medicine. *Authors*: Lam, Y., Luft, B. J., Litcher-Kelly, L., Shaw, R. D., Bucobo, J. C., Bromet, E., Kotov, R., Banker, S. V., Brand, D. L., Broihier, J. A., *Record Number*: 3294, *Pages*: 686–93 *Volume*: 76 *Number*: 9 *Edition*: November 07, 2014

World Trade Center disaster exposure-related probable posttraumatic stress disorder among responders and civilians: a meta-analysis, PloS One, *Authors*: Kim, H., Bromet, E. J., Liu, B., Tarigan, L. H., *Record Number*: 3075, *Pages*: e101491 *Volume*: 9 *Number*: 7 *Edition*: July 23, 2014

Post-disaster stressful life events and WTC-related posttraumatic stress, depressive symptoms, and overall functioning among responders to the World Trade Center disaster, Journal of Psychiatric Research, *Authors*: Vujanovic, A., Reissman, D. B., Gonzalez, A., Udasin, I., Crane, M., Pietrzak, R. H., Luft, B. J., Kaplan, J., Zvolensky, M. J., Moline, J., Kotov, R., Southwick, S. M., Schechter, C. B., Feder, A. *Record Number*:3270, *Edition*: December 17, 2014

Bromet, E. J., Moline, J., Kotov, R., Kaplan, J., Luft, B. J., Guerrera, K., Von Korff, M., Gonzalez, A., Udasin, I., Schechter, C., Pietrzak, R. H., Broihier, J., Reissman, D., Feder, A., Ruggero, C., Friedman-Jimenez, G., Southwick, S. M. *Posttraumatic stress disorder and the risk of respiratory problems in World Trade Center responders: longitudinal test of a pathway*, Psychosomatic Medicine, *Record Number*:3301, *Edition*: April 29, 2015

Schechter, C. B., Southwick, S. M., Kotov, R., Moline, J., Farris, S. G., Kaplan, J., Zvolensky, M. J., Crane, M., Bromet, E., Feder, A., Gonzalez, A., Udasin, I., Vujanovic, A., Reissman, D. B., Pietrzak, R. H., Luft, B. J. *World Trade Center disaster and sensitization to subsequent life stress: a longitudinal study of disaster responders*, Preventive Medicine *Pages*: 70–74, *Volume*: 75 *Edition*: April 04, 2015

Conclusion

The WTC disaster has led to an innovative medical screening and treatment program, providing needed care to the men and women who responded when the United States was attacked on September 11, 2001. Not only did we see the heroism that ensued, but it has furthered medical understanding of diseases like sarcoidosis, and provided unique insights into the physical manifestations of illness after a large disaster. The information gathered from the medical programs developed in the years after September 11 have been informative, and, through the Zadroga Act, research will continue into the years to come. This valuable cohort of exposed individuals will teach us not only about bravery and perseverance, but also the long-term sequelae of a massive disaster.

References

1. Pleil JD, Vette AF, Johnson BA, Rappaport SM. Air levels of carcinogenic polycyclic aromatic hydrocarbons after the World Trade Center disaster. Proc Natl Acad Sci U S A. 2004;101:11685–8.
2. Lioy PJ, Weisel CP, Millette JR, Eisenreich S, Vallero D, Offenberg J, Buckley B, Turpin B, Zhong M, Cohen MD, Prophete C, Yang I, Stiles R, Chee G, Johnson W, Porcja R, Alimokhtari S, Hale RC, Weschler C, Chen LC. Characterization of the dust/smoke aerosol that settled east of the World Trade Center (WTC) in lower Manhattan after the collapse of the WTC 11 September 2001. Environ Health Perspect. 2002;10:703–14.
3. McGee JK, Chen LC, Cohen MD, Chee GR, Prophete CM, Haykal-Coates N, Wasson SJ, Conner TL, Costa DL, Gavett SH. Chemical analysis of World Trade Center fine particulate matter for use in toxicologic assessment. Environ Health Perspect. 2003;111:972–80.
4. EPA, U. S. Exposure and human health evaluation of airborne pollution from the World Trade Center disaster – external review draft. Washington, DC: U.S. Environmental Protection Agency; 2002.
5. CDC. Occupational exposures to air contaminants at the World Trade Center disaster site – New York, September-October, 2001. MMWR Morb Mortal Wkly Rep. 2002;51:453–6.
6. Banauch G, Dhala A, Prezant D. Pulmonary disease in rescue workers at the World Trade Center site. Curr Opin Pulm Med. 2005;11:160–8.
7. EPA, U. S. Toxicological effects of fine particulate matter derived from the destruction of the World Trade Center. Research Triangle Park, NC: U.S. Environmental Protection Agency; 2002.
8. Jeffrey N, D'andrea C, Leighton J, Rodenbeck S, Wilder L, Devoney D, Neurath S, Lee C, Williams R. Potential exposures to airborne and settled surface dust in residential areas of lower Manhattan following the collapse of the World Trade Center – New York City, November 4–December 11, 2001. Morb Mortal Wkly Rep. 2003;52:131–6.
9. Offenberg JH, Eisenreich SJ, Gigliotti CL, Chen LC, Xiong JQ, Quan C, Xiaopeng L, Zhong M, Gorczynski J, Yiin L-M, Illacqua V, Lioy PJ. Persistent organic pollutants in dusts that settled indoors in lower Manhattan after September 11, 2001. J Expo Anal Environ Epidemiol. 2004;14:164–72.
10. Service, R. World Trade Center. Chemical studies of 9/11 disaster tell complex tale of 'bad stuff'. Science. 2003;301:1649.
11. Wallingford KM, Snyder EM. Occupational exposures during the World Trade Center disaster response. Toxicol Ind Health. 2001;17:247–53.

12. Fireman EM, Lerman Y, Ganor E, Greif J, Fireman-Shoresh S, Lioy PJ, Banauch GI, Weiden M, Kelly KJ, Prezant DJ. Induced sputum assessment in New York City firefighters exposed to World Trade Center dust. Environ Health Perspect. 2004;112:1564–9.
13. Herbert R, Moline J, Skloot GS, Metzger K, Baron S, Luft B, Markowitz S, Udasin I, Harrison D, Stein D, Todd AC, Enright P, Mager Stellman J, Landrigan PJ, Levin S. The World Trade Center disaster and the health of workers: five-year assessment of a unique medical screening program. Environ Health Perspect. 2006;114:1853–8.
14. Levin S, Herbert R, Skloot GS, Szeinuk J, Teirstein AS, Fischler D, Milek D, Piligian G, Wilk-Rivard E, Moline J. Health effects of World Trade Center site workers. Am J Ind Med. 2002;42:545–7.
15. Prezant DJ, Weiden M, Banauch GI, McGuinness G, Rom WN, Aldrich TK, Kelly KJ. Cough and bronchial responsiveness in firefighters at the World Trade Center site. N Engl J Med. 2002;347:806–15.
16. Mann JM, Sha KK, Kline G, Breuer FU, Miller A. World Trade Center dyspnea: bronchiolitis obliterans with functional improvement: a case report. Am J Ind Med. 2005;48:225–9.
17. Rom WN, Weiden M, Garcia R, Yie TA, Vathesatogkit P, Tse DB, McGuinness G, Roggli V, Prezant D. Acute eosinophilic pneumonia in a New York City firefighter exposed to World Trade Center dust. Am J Respir Crit Care Med. 2002;166:797–800.
18. Safirstein BH, Klukowicz A, Miller R, Teirstein A. Granulomatous pneumonitis following exposure to the World Trade Center collapse. Chest. 2003;123:301–4.
19. CDC. Physical health status of World Trade Center rescue and recovery workers and volunteers – New York City, July 2002–August 2004. MMWR Morb Mortal Wkly Rep. 2004;53:807–12.
20. Moline JM, Herbert R, Crowley LE, Troy K, Hodgman E, Shukla G, Udasin I, Luft BJ, Wallenstein S, Landrigan P, Savitz DA. Multiple myeloma in World Trade Center responders: a case series. J Occup Environ Med. 2009;51:896–902.
21. James Zadroga 9/11 Health and Compensation Act of 2010.
22. Lioy PJ, Gochfeld M. Lessons learned on environmental, occupational, and residential exposures from the attack on the World Trade Center. Am J Ind Med. 2002;42:560–5.
23. USGS. U.S. Geological Survey open file report OFR-01-0429. Environmental studies of the World Trade Center area after the September 11, 2001 attack. Reston: U.S. Geological Survey; 2002.
24. Lioy PJ, Weisel CP, Millette JR, Eisenreich S, Vallero D, Offenberg J, Buckley B, Turpin B, Zhong M, Cohen MD, Prophete C, Yang I, Stiles R, Chee G, Johnson W, Porcja R, Alimokhtari S, Hale RC, Weschler C, Chen LC. Characterization of the dust/smoke aerosol that settled east of the World Trade Center (WTC) in lower Manhattan after the collapse of the WTC 11 September 2001. Environ Health Perspect. 2002;110:703–14.
25. Gavett SH, Haykal-Coates N, Highfill JW, Ledbetter AD, Chen LC, Cohen MD, Harkema JR, Wagner JG, Costa DL. World Trade Center fine particulate matter causes respiratory tract hyperresponsiveness in mice. Environ Health Perspect. 2003;111:981–91.
26. Prezant DJ. World Trade Center Cough Syndrome and its treatment. Lung. 2008;186(Suppl 1): S94–102.
27. Wisnivesky JP, Teitelbaum SL, Todd AC, Boffetta P, Crane M, Crowley L, De la Hoz RE, Dellenbaugh C, Harrison D, Herbert R, Kim H, Jeon Y, Kaplan J, Katz CL, Levin S, Luft B, Markowitz S, Moline J, Ozbay F, Pietrzak RH, Shapiro M, Sharma V, Skloot GS, Southwick S, Stevenson LA, Udasin I, Wallenstein S, Landrigan P. Persistence of multiple illnesses in World Trade Center rescue and recovery workers: a cohort study. Lancet. 2011;378:888–97.
28. Izbicki G, Chavko R, Banauch GI, Weiden MD, Berger KI, Aldrich TK, Hall C, Kelly KJ, Prezant DJ. World Trade Center "sarcoid-like" granulomatous pulmonary disease in New York City Fire Department rescue workers. Chest. 2007;131:1414–23.
29. Jordan HT, Stellman SD, Prezant DJ, Teirstein AS, Osahan SS, Cone JE. Sarcoidosis diagnosed after September 11, 2001 among adults exposed to the World Trade Center disaster. J Occup Environ Med. 2011;53:966–74.

30. Crowley LE, Herbert R, Moline JM, Wallenstein S, Shukla G, Schechter CB, Skloot GS, Udasin I, Luft BJ, Harrison D, Shapiro M, Wong K, Sacks HS, Landrigan PJ, Teirstein AS. "Sarcoid like" granulomatous pulmonary disease in World Trade Center disaster responders. Am J Ind Med. 2011;54:175–84.

31. Skloot GS, Schechter CB, Herbert R, Moline JM, Levin SM, Crowley LE, Luft BJ, Udasin IG, Enright PL. Longitudinal assessment of spirometry in the World Trade Center medical monitoring program. Chest. 2009;135:492–8.

32. Berger KI, Reibman J, Oppenheimer BW, Vlahos I, Harrison D, Goldring RM. Lessons from the World Trade Center Disaster: airway disease presenting as restrictive dysfunction. Chest. 2013;144:249–57.

33. Friedman SM, Maslow CB, Reibman J, Pillai PS, Goldring RM, Farfel MR, Stellman SD, Berger KI. Case-control study of lung function in World Trade Center Health Registry area residents and workers. Am J Respir Crit Care Med. 2011;184:582–9.

34. Banauch GI, Hall C, Weiden M, Cohen HW, Aldrich TK, Christodoulou V, Arcentales N, Kelly KJ, Prezant DJ. Pulmonary function after exposure to the World Trade Center collapse in the New York City Fire Department. Am J Respir Crit Care Med. 2006;174:312–9.

35. Aldrich TK, Gustave J, Hall C, Cohen HW, Webber MP, Zeig-Owens R, Cosenza K, Christodoulou V, Glass L, Al-Othman F, Weiden M, Kelly KJ, Prezant DJ. Lung function in rescue workers at the World Trade Center after 7 years. N Engl J Med. 2010;362:1263–72.

36. Weiden M, Ferrier N, Nolan A, Rom W, Comfort A, Gustave J, Zeig-Owens R, Zheng S, Goldring R, Berger K, Cosenza K, Lee R, Webber M, Kelly K, Aldrich T, Prezant D. Obstructive airways disease with air trapping among firefighters exposed to World Trade Center dust. Chest. 2010;137:566–74.

37. Banauch GI, Brantly M, Izbicki G, Hall C, Shanske A, Chauko R, Santhyadka G, Christodoulou V, Weiden MD, Prezant DJ. Accelerated spirometric decline in New York City firefighters with alpha1-antitrypsin deficiency. Chest. 2010;138:1116–24.

38. Salzman SH, Moosavy FM, Miskoff JA, Friedmann P, Fried G, Rosen MJ. Early respiratory abnormalities in emergency services police officers at the World Trade Center site. J Occup Environ Med. 2004;46:113–22.

39. Skloot G, Goldman M, Fischler D, Goldman C, Schechter C, Levin S, Teirstein A. Respiratory symptoms and physiologic assessment of ironworkers at the World Trade Center disaster site. Chest. 2004;125:1248–55.

40. Oppenheimer B, Goldring R, Herberg M, Hofer I, Reyfman P, Liautaud S, Rom W, Reibman J, Berger K. Distal airway function in symptomatic subjects with normal spirometry following World Trade Center dust exposure. Chest. 2007;132:1275–82.

41. Solan S, Wallenstein S, Shapiro M, Teitelbaum S, Stevenson L, Kochman A, Kaplan J, Dellenbaugh C, Kahn A, Biro F, Crane M, Crowley L, Gabrilove J, Gonsalves L, Harrison D, Herbert R, Luft B, Markowitz S, Moline J, Niu X, Sacks H, Shukla G, Udasin I, Lucchini R, Boffetta P, Landrigan P. Cancer incidence in World Trade Center rescue and recovery workers, 2001-2008. Environ Health Perspect. 2013;121:699–704.

42. Zeig-Owens R, Webber MP, Hall C, Schwartz T, Jaber N, Weakley J, Rohan TE, Cohen HW, Derman O, Aldrich TK, Kelly KJ, Prezant DJ. Early assessment of cancer outcomes in New York City firefighters after the 9/11 attacks: an observational cohort study. Lancet. 2011;378:898–905.

43. Department of Health and Human Services, U. S. 42 CFR part 88 – World Trade Center health program requirements for the addition of new WTC-related health conditions. Washington, D.C.: Department of Health and Human Services; 2012.

44. CDC 2015. WTC Health Program Research-to-Care Logic Model. 1–5. From the WTC health program steering committee; 2015.

45. Moline J, Herbert R, Nguyen N. Health consequences of the September 11 World Trade Center attacks: a review. Cancer Investig. 2006;24:294–301.

46. Nolan RP, Ross M, Nord GL, Axten CW, Osleeb JP, Domnin SG, Bertram P, Wilson R. Risk assessment for asbestos-related cancer from the 9/11 attack on the World Trade Center. J Occup Med. 2005;47:817–25.

47. Rayne S. Using exterior building surface films to assess human exposure and health risks from PCDD/Fs in New York City, USA, after the World Trade Center attacks. J Hazard Mater. 2005;127:33–9.

48. Samet JM, Geyh AS, Utell MJ. The legacy of World Trade Center dust. N Engl J Med. 2007;356:2233–6.

49. World Trade Center Health Program Research Projects [Online]. WTC Health Program Research Gateway. 2016. Available: https://wwwn.cdc.gov/ResearchGateway/ResearchProjects. Accessed 7 Nov 2016.

Long-Term PTSD and Comorbidity with Depression Among World Trade Center Responders

Evelyn J. Bromet, Roman Kotov, and Benjamin J. Luft

Abbreviations

DSM-IV	*Diagnostic and Statistical Manual of Mental Disorders 4th edition*
FDNY-WTC-MMP	Fire Department of the City of New York World Trade Center Medical Monitoring Program
MDD	Major depressive disorder
NIOSH	National Institute of Occupational Safety and Health
PCL	Posttraumatic Symptom Checklist
PTSD	Posttraumatic stress disorder
RIFT	Range of Impaired Functioning Tool
SCID	Structured Clinical Interview for DSM-IV
WTC	World Trade Center
WTC-HP	World Trade Center Health Program
WTC-HR	World Trade Center Health Registry

Introduction

Responders to the World Trade Center (WTC) disaster were exposed to emotional horrors and complex environmental toxins from gases and fine airborne particulate matter. The ~90,000 responders included trained first responders

E.J. Bromet (✉) • R. Kotov
Department of Psychiatry, Stony Brook University, Stony Brook, NY 11794, USA
e-mail: bromet@stonybrookmedicine.edu; Roman.kotov@stonybrook.edu

B.J. Luft
Department of Medicine, Stony Brook University, Stony Brook, NY 11794, USA
e-mail: Benjamin.Luft@stonybrook.edu

© Springer International Publishing AG 2018   21
A.M. Szema (ed.), *World Trade Center Pulmonary Diseases
and Multi-Organ System Manifestations*, DOI 10.1007/978-3-319-59372-2_2

(e.g., police and firefighters) and inexperienced nontraditional responders, such as construction workers, electricians, and transportation and utility workers [1]. In the aftermath of the tower collapse, three large-scale health monitoring programs were funded by the National Institute of Occupational Safety and Health (NIOSH): the Fire Department of the City of New York Medical Monitoring Program (FDNY-WTC-MMP); and the WTC Health Program (WTC-HP) established for police, other non-FDNY professionals, and nontraditional rescue/cleanup/recovery workers at five coordinated centers of excellence (Mount Sinai School of Medicine, Stony Brook University, Bellevue/New York University, Queens College, and Rutgers Robert Wood Johnson Medical School); and the WTC Health Registry (WTC-HR) which conducts longitudinal surveys of exposed civilians and responders.

The FDNY-WTC-MMP and WTC-HP provide ongoing assessments of both physical and mental health from direct physical examinations and self-report questionnaires and also treat WTC-related conditions. The WTC-HR collects survey data on physical and mental health. It is important to note that these programs are the first known health surveillance programs established after a toxic disaster that evaluate both physical and mental health, rather than solely focusing on physical outcomes.

This chapter focuses on posttraumatic stress disorder (PTSD) among responders. PTSD is a condition that can arise soon after a traumatic event (although symptoms may appear or become impairing after months or years have passed). The *Diagnostic and Statistical Manual of Mental Disorders 4th edition* (DSM-IV) organized PTSD symptoms into three clusters: reexperiencing symptoms (e.g., intrusive recollections, nightmares, flashbacks), avoidance and numbing symptoms (e.g., avoiding reminders of the event, feeling detached, sense of foreshortened future), and hyperarousal symptoms (e.g., difficulty falling or staying asleep, irritability, difficulty concentrating, hypervigilance, exaggerated startle response). The diagnosis is made only when a sufficient number of symptoms in each category co-occur, last longer than a month, and interfere with a person's functioning.

Because PTSD was the most common mental health condition being studied in disaster research, each of the three large-scale monitoring programs has assessed PTSD since 2002, when they were established. The assessment instrument used by all three programs is the Posttraumatic Symptom Checklist (PCL), a 17-item self-report measure designed to assess the severity of the PTSD symptoms listed in DSM-IV [2] over the past month on a scale from 1 (not at all) to 5 (extremely). Scores can range from very low (17) to very high (85). Numerous WTC publications have described the prevalence of probable PTSD based on PCL cut points of either 44 or 50 or a proxy DSM-based PTSD measure created from the requisite number of moderate to severe symptoms in each of the three clusters (reexperiencing, avoidance, and hyperarousal).

Prevalence of PTSD in WTC Responders

The first paper on probable PTSD in WTC-HP responders examined more than 10,000 participants whose first monitoring visit occurred within 5 years of the attack [3]. Eleven percent met criteria for probable PTSD, a rate the authors described as similar to the rate in US veterans returning from Afghanistan. The rate is also almost three times higher than the rate of PTSD among men in the general population who reported being exposed to a traumatic event (4.1%; [4]). Stellman et al. also found that PTSD decreased across the 5 years of observation (2002–2006), but a study of FDNY using data from the same period of time found the reverse, namely, that the rate of probable PTSD increased during that period [5]. In addition to the early reports from the WTC-HP and FDNY programs, a number of reports on probable PTSD were published by the WTC-HR. The latter confirmed the high rate of PTSD in responders and also reported significantly more PTSD in nontraditional compared to police responders [6], a pattern also observed in WTC-HP participants [7]. Subsequently, Pietrzak et al. [8] conducted trajectory analyses using PCL data from WTC-HP responders' three initial monitoring visits and found that 5.3% of police and 9.5% of nontraditional responders had chronically elevated symptom levels. The data from all three large monitoring programs were consistent in reporting that exposure severity, defined by variables such as death of colleagues, early arrival at the site (September 11 to September 12), injuries, and relatively long duration of work, was significantly associated with an increased rate of PTSD.

A few studies evaluated the long-term prevalence of probable PTSD more than a decade after 9/11. Cone et al. [9] analyzed data from police enrolled in the WTC-HR and found that 11% had probable PTSD at 10–11-year follow-up, half of whom also had PTSD at earlier time points. Thus, even more than a decade after 9/11, in men who were previously considered "a healthy worker" cohort and indeed were screened for resilience prior to entry into the police academy, the rate of long-term, probable PTSD was more than double that of an unselected sample of men in the general population who reported trauma exposure.

To date, only four studies of WTC-PTSD in responders have been based on actual clinical diagnostic interviews rather than the PCL. A clinical interview allows a professional rater to probe for all DSM-IV criteria, symptoms, duration, and impairment. Two studies administered the Clinician-Administered PTSD Scale [10], which is considered the gold standard for assessment of PTSD. The first study assessed mental health relief workers 6–8 months after 9/11; 6.4% met developed WTC-related PTSD [11]. The second was a longitudinal study of utility workers that reported a decline in PTSD from 15% in 2002 to 5% in 2008 [12]. The Diagnostic Interview Schedule was administered to a large sample of retired firefighters 5–6 years after 9/11; 7% of the sample had active PTSD [13]. The fourth study was conducted at the Stony Brook WTC-HP and involved an assessment of

~3500 responders in 2012–2014 using the Structured Clinical Interview for DSM-IV (SCID; [14]). Eighteen percent developed WTC-PTSD during that period, and 10% had current PTSD at the time of interview. Consistent with the PCL findings, the rates were higher in nontraditional than police responders and were significantly associated with severity of exposure (early arrival, longer hours of work, exposure to the dust cloud).

Comorbidity of PTSD and Physical Health

A large number of studies have shown strong reciprocal and longitudinal associations of PTSD with several aspects of physical health, particularly respiratory (e.g., [7, 15]) and gastrointestinal [16, 17] conditions. The Stony Brook studies in particular [7, 15] showed that PTSD was not just a correlate but was a significant driver of lower respiratory symptoms, with new onsets being twice as common and recovery being half as common in responders with PTSD at their previous visit compared to responders free from PTSD. This finding was consistent with evidence of a biological pathway between these conditions. As shown in Fig. 1, the pathway also includes poor health behaviors, such as smoking and substance abuse.

Indeed, it is important to note that PTSD has consistently been tied to neurohormonal dysregulation in stress response systems (e.g., [18]), including sympathetic hyperactivity [19] and altered hypothalamic-pituitary-adrenal (HPA) axis functioning [18]. The latter has been reflected in low peripheral cortisol at rest, increased suppression during pharmacological challenge paradigm, and increased cortisol reactivity following cognitive challenge. Dysfunction in both sympathetic and HPA systems is known to be associated with increased levels of pro-inflammatory cytokines (e.g., interleukin-1 and interleukin-6) (e.g., [20]). Of note, immunologic dysregulation has been documented across several studies of PTSD. These inflammatory

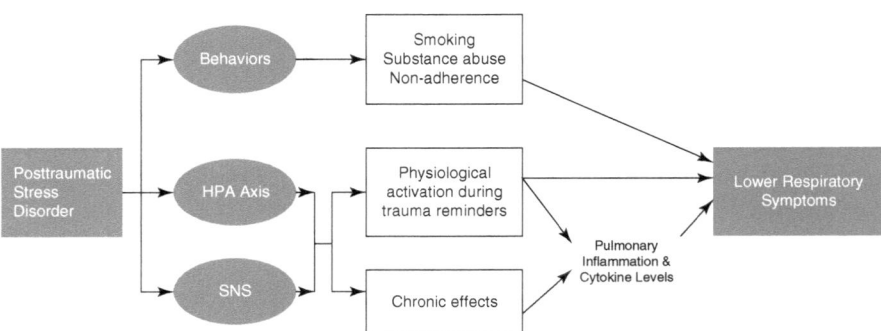

¹Modified from Vaccarino and Bremner, 2013

Fig. 1 Pathways between PTSD and lower respiratory symptoms. Modified from Vaccarino and Bremner [26]

processes in turn may contribute to medical comorbidities, including respiratory illnesses, as observed in the Stony Brook responder cohort [15].

In addition to associations between PTSD and physical health, a recent study showed that PTSD, especially the reexperiencing symptom cluster, was also predictive of cognitive impairment 14 years after 9/11 [21]. Recent studies of veterans have also shown associations between PTSD and cognitive impairment, but a large proportion of veteran samples has comorbid traumatic brain injuries, making it difficult to disentangle the effects of PTSD from those of traumatic brain injury. While the results from the Stony Brook study need to be replicated, if confirmed, they suggest that the consequences of persistent PTSD reach beyond the medical symptoms that have been the focus of most of the WTC research to date. They also raise questions about potential changes in the brain resulting from chronic and persistent PTSD.

The findings on PTSD in WTC responders have been consistent with 50 years of research showing that mental ill health is associated with disability, physical morbidity, and even mortality. Thus, treating PTSD in WTC responders and survivors is a priority for WTC health programs as well as society more generally. The most commonly prescribed medications are antidepressants, and the most common forms of psychotherapy are psychoeducation, exposure therapy, and cognitive behavioral therapy. However, it has been estimated that the majority of individuals with PTSD either improve slowly or fail to improve after various medication and psychotherapy trials. Thus, in light of the protracted nature of PTSD, the need for care remains a continuing challenge.

Comorbidity of PTSD and Major Depression

Many clinical- and population-based studies have shown that PTSD and major depressive disorder are significantly comorbid and that this is particularly true for chronic PTSD, as shown in several WTC PCL-based studies (e.g., [9, 22, 23]) and diagnosis-based research [14]. In the Stony Brook study of 3504 responders, 204 responders met diagnostic criteria for *both* current DSM-IV PTSD and current major depressive disorder (MDD) 11–13 years after 9/11. This represented almost half (47.7%) of responders with either one of these disorders ($N = 428$; odds ratio = 1.42; 95% confidence interval = 1.43–1.53; $p = 0.000$). For the remainder of the chapter, we explore whether responders with current comorbid PTSD/MDD were significantly more disadvantaged with regard to their health and quality of life than responders with single or with no current disorder.

Specifically, we compared three groups: responders with current DSM-IV PTSD/MDD, responders with either PTSD or MDD, and responders with neither condition (Table 1). We first compared them on demographic characteristics. In the three-way comparison, the groups were similar in age at the time of 9/11 but differed significantly on sex, occupational and marital status, and police versus nontraditional responder status. That is, the comorbid PTSD/MDD group contained the largest

Table 1 Comparison of Stony Brook WTC Health Program responders with current comorbid PTSD and MDD, single disorder, and neither

	Neither N = 3076	Single disorder N = 224	Current PTSD/MDD N = 204	
	%	%	%	p
Demographics				
Age in 2001, 40+	39.8	37.5	46.6	NS
Sex, female	8.1	12.9	14.2	***
Currently not working	26.4	55.9	65.2	***
Currently not married	12.0	15.6	21.1	***
Nontraditional responder	25.4	42.4	46.6	***
WTC experiences				
Lost co-workers/colleagues	66.9	74.5	77.1	**
Exposed to the dust cloud	22.5	25.1	28.2	NS
WTC lower respiratory condition	39.5	69.5	74.9	***
Diagnosed with a WTC condition	44.2	68.3	81.9	***
Quality of life				
Rate their health as poor	5.6	24.2	39.1	***
Poor life satisfaction	29.5	63.7	83.3	***
Poor relationships with friends	16.8	37.1	52.4	***
Inadequate social support	28.4	58.0	63.1	***

NS not significant, * $p \leq 0.05$, ** $p \leq 0.01$, *** $p \leq 0.001$

proportion of women, unmarried and unemployed responders, and those coming from nontraditional occupations, while the group with neither condition contained the fewest responders who were female, unmarried, out of the workforce, or in the nontraditional responder category. The single-disorder group fell in between. Of note, two-thirds of responders with PTSD/MDD were out of the workforce compared to ~50% in the single-disorder group and one-quarter in the group having neither disorder. The two-way comparisons of responders in the PTSD/MDD versus single-disorder groups indicated a trend for those with both disorders to be older ($p = 0.057$) and not in the workforce ($p = 0.052$).

Regarding WTC experiences, we analyzed two key exposures and two key health effects. With regard to exposures, the three groups did not differ significantly on dust cloud exposure. However, three-quarters of responders with single and with comorbid PTSD/MDD lost colleagues and friends when the towers collapsed compared to two-thirds of responders with neither disorder ($p = 0.002$). In terms of WTC health effects, responders with neither PTSD nor MDD were the least, and comorbid PTSD/MDD responders the most, likely to have current lower respiratory symptoms and to report that they were told by a doctor that they have a WTC-related condition. In the no-disorder group, 44.2% reported that they were diagnosed with a WTC-related condition. In contrast, among responders with comorbid PTSD/MDD, 81.9% reported such a diagnosis. In the single-disorder group, the figure was 68.3% (p value for the two-way comparison = 0.003).

We next examined health-related quality of life (self-rated health as poor or very poor on a five-point scale) and impairments in life satisfaction, relationships with friends, and adequacy of social support. The latter three domains were determined from the Range of Impaired Functioning Tool (RIFT) developed by Leon et al. [24]. These domains represent interviewer ratings made after a series of probes on a five-point scale from very positive to very negative. Impairment scores for each scale were dichotomized as follows: life satisfaction (fair/poor/very poor versus good/very good), impaired friendships (mild/moderate/severe impairment versus satisfactory/non-impaired friendships), and social support (fair/poor social network involvement versus good/very good).

As shown in Table 1, each of the three-way comparisons was highly significant, with the no-disorder group having the lowest and the comorbid group the highest percent reporting poor subjective health and rated as having impairment in each domain. Indeed, four out of five comorbid responders had impaired life satisfaction, and two out of three had inadequate social support. The rank ordering across the three groups was particularly striking. The two-way comparison further indicated that significantly more comorbid responders had poor subjective health ratings and impaired functioning compared to responders with a single disorder ($p \leq 0.001$).

Conclusion

WTC experiences have taken an enduring toll on responders. Fortunately, there are programs in place to monitor and treat their physical and mental health conditions. Comorbid PTSD/MDD has proven to be a particularly severe mental health outcome, having an adverse association with not just physical health but also quality of life. One surprising finding was that although nontraditional responders are at increased risk of long-term PTSD and MDD, there was no difference by responder status in the rate of comorbid PTSD/MDD. In general, the findings from the published literature and from this secondary analysis of comorbid PTSD/MDD 11–13 years after 9/11 showed that half of responders with long-term PTSD also had comorbid MDD and comorbidity was associated with multiple forms of impairment many years after 9/11, including being out of the workforce and having poor life satisfaction. These results confirm earlier findings based on the PCL [23] and support the need for continued screening and treatment of both PTSD and MDD and comorbid PTSD/MDD.

Since the bombings in Japan in 1945, a number of toxic disasters have occurred, ranging from the gas leak at Bhopal primarily from methyl isocyanate (1984), to the vast radiation contamination from the explosion at the Chernobyl nuclear power plant (1986), to the sarin attack on the Tokyo subway (1995), and to the triple disaster in Fukushima which led to the evacuation of 220,000 residents living in the 20–30 km area near the Daiichi plants (2011). Each event had both physical and mental health consequences. Yet only after the WTC attacks were both physical and mental health evaluated concurrently. After the Fukushima radiation disaster, self-report health questionnaires were mailed to evacuees and other affected populations, and self-report mental health and lifestyle questionnaires were also posted. But they were done as separate mailings. After the three nuclear power plant accidents (Three Mile Island, Chernobyl, Fukushima), the consensus reports issued by the major international radiation agencies all concluded that the biggest public health impact of these events was on mental health. Yet in spite of the 1948 World Health Organization statement that health encompasses physical, mental, and social well-being, and in spite of the research findings on mental health after these large-scale toxic disasters, mental health was not viewed as a direct effect and hence did not fall within the purview of health monitoring and research programs, even as a risk factor. It is well established that mental and physical health are two sides of the same coin, each influencing the other, with mental health in some instances serving as the driver of physical morbidity and mortality. The fact that the WTC monitoring programs assess and offer treatment for both aspects of health has been a momentous step forward.

Since the first epidemiologic evidence on PTSD [25], the chronicity of PTSD has been well known. Furthermore, the original study by Kessler, the National Comorbidity Survey, showed that respondents with a history of untreated PTSD had a longer course of illness than those who had sought treatment. PTSD is one of the most difficult disorders to treat effectively, in part because of its complexity and in part because of its comorbidity with other disorders, including depression described in this chapter but also substance abuse and other anxiety disorders. Nonetheless, some treatments, such as exposure therapy and antidepressants, are effective for some individuals. Although treatment often proceeds by trial and error, it is reasonable to hope that an effective treatment can be found for responders with PTSD, even if initiated long after its onset. Short of that, long-term support from clinical staff in programs such as the Stony Brook WTC-HP and certification of PTSD and depression, which allows for treatment without charge to the responders, minimize the sense of isolation and unhappiness that arise in individuals with chronic mental disorders.

References

1. Dasaro CR, Holden WL, Berman KD, Crane MA, Kaplan JR, Lucchini RG, et al. Cohort profile: World Trade Center Health Program general responder cohort. Int J Epidemiol. 2015 10.1093/ije/dyv099. Epub.
2. Blanchard EB, Jones-Alexander J, Buckley TC, Forneris CA. Psychometric properties of the PTSD Checklist (PCL). Behav Res Ther. 1996;34(8):669–73.
3. Stellman JM, Smith RP, Katz CL, Sharma V, Charney DS, Herbert R, et al. Enduring mental health morbidity and social function impairment in world trade center rescue, recovery, and cleanup workers: the psychological dimension of an environmental health disaster. Environ Health Perspect. 2008;116(9):1248–53.
4. Pietrzak RH, Goldstein RB, Southwick SM, Grant BF. Prevalence and Axis I comorbidity of full and partial posttraumatic stress disorder in the United States: results from Wave 2 of

the National Epidemiologic Survey on Alcohol and Related Conditions. J Anxiety Disord. 2011;25(3):456–65.

5. Berninger A, Webber MP, Cohen HW, Gustave J, Lee R, Niles JK, et al. Trends of elevated PTSD risk in firefighters exposed to the World Trade Center disaster: 2001–2005. Public Health Rep. 2010;125(4):556–66.

6. Perrin MA, DiGrande L, Wheeler K, Thorpe L, Farfel M, Brackbill R. Differences in PTSD prevalence and associated risk factors among World Trade Center disaster rescue and recovery workers. Am J Psychiatry. 2007;164(9):1385–94.

7. Luft BJ, Schechter C, Kotov R, Broihier J, Reissman D, Guerrera K, et al. Exposure, probable PTSD and lower respiratory illness among World Trade Center rescue, recovery and clean-up workers. Psychol Med. 2012;42(5):1069–79.

8. Pietrzak RH, Feder A, Singh R, Schechter CB, Bromet EJ, Katz CL, et al. Trajectories of PTSD risk and resilience in World Trade Center responders: an 8-year prospective cohort study. Psychol Med. 2014;44(1):205–19.

9. Cone JE, Li J, Kornblith E, Gocheva V, Stellman SD, Shaikh A, Schwarzer R, et al. Chronic probable PTSD in police responders in the world trade center health registry ten to eleven years after 9/11. Am J Ind Med. 2015;58(5):483–93.

10. Blake DD, Weathers FW, Nagy LM, Kaloupek DG, Gusman FD, Charney DS, et al. The development of a Clinician-Administered PTSD Scale. J Trauma Stress. 1995;8(1):75–90.

11. Zimering R, Gulliver SB, Knight J, Munroe J, Keane TM. Posttraumatic stress disorder in disaster relief workers following direct and indirect trauma exposure to Ground Zero. J Trauma Stress. 2006;19(4):553–7.

12. Cukor J, Wyka K, Mello B, Olden M, Jayasinghe N, Roberts J, et al. The longitudinal course of PTSD among disaster workers deployed to the World Trade Center following the attacks of September 11th. J Trauma Stress. 2011;24(5):506–14.

13. Chiu S, Webber MP, Zeig-Owens R, Gustave J, Lee R, Kelly KJ, et al. Performance characteristics of the PTSD Checklist in retired firefighters exposed to the World Trade Center disaster. Ann Clin Psychiatry. 2011;23(2):95–104.

14. Bromet EJ, Hobbs MJ, Clouston SA, Gonzalez A, Kotov R, Luft BJ. DSM-IV post-traumatic stress disorder among World Trade Center responders 11–13 years after the disaster of 11 September 2001 (9/11). Psychol Med. 2016;46(4):771–83.

15. Kotov R, Bromet EJ, Schechter C, Broihier J, Feder A, Friedman-Jimenez G, et al. Posttraumatic stress disorder and the risk of respiratory problems in World Trade Center responders: longitudinal test of a pathway. Psychosom Med. 2015;77(4):438–48.

16. Litcher-Kelly L, Lam Y, Broihier JA, Brand DL, Banker SV, Kotov R, et al. Longitudinal study of the impact of psychological distress symptoms on new-onset upper gastrointestinal symptoms in World Trade Center responders. Psychosom Med. 2014;76(9):686–93.

17. Wisnivesky JP, Teitelbaum SL, Todd AC, Boffetta P, Crane M, Crowley L, et al. Persistence of multiple illnesses in World Trade Center rescue and recovery workers: a cohort study. Lancet. 2011;378(9794):888–97.

18. Yehuda R. Status of glucocorticoid alterations in post-traumatic stress disorder. Ann N Y Acad Sci. 2009;1179:56–69.

19. Pole N. The psychophysiology of posttraumatic stress disorder: a meta-analysis. Psychol Bull. 2007;133(5):725–46.

20. Spitzer C, Barnow S, Völzke H, Wallaschofski H, John U, Freyberger HJ, et al. Association of posttraumatic stress disorder with low-grade elevation of C-reactive protein: evidence from the general population. J Psychiatr Res. 2010;44(1):15–21.

21. Clouston SA, Kotov R, Pietrzak RH, Luft BJ, Gonzalez A, Richards M, et al. Cognitive impairment among World Trade Center responders: Long-term implications of re-experiencing the 9/11 terrorist attacks. Alzheimers Dement (Amsterdam). 2016;19(4):67–75.

22. Bowler RM, Kornblith ES, Li J, Adams SW, Gocheva VV, Schwarzer R, et al. Police officers who responded to 9/11: comorbidity of PTSD, depression, and anxiety 10–11 years later. Am J Ind Med. 2016;59(6):425–36.

23. Caramanica K, Brackbill RM, Liao T, Stellman SD. Comorbidity of 9/11-related PTSD and depression in the World Trade Center Health Registry 10–11 years postdisaster. J Trauma Stress. 2014;27(6):680–8.
24. Leon AC, Solomon DA, Mueller TI, Turvey CL, Endicott J, Keller MB. The range of impaired functioning tool (LIFE-RIFT): a brief measure of functional impairment. Psychol Med. 1999;29(4):869–78.
25. Kessler RC, Sonnega A, Bromet E, Hughes M, Nelson CB. Posttraumatic stress disorder in the National Comorbidity Survey. Arch Gen Psychiatry. 1995;52(12):1048–60.
26. Vaccarino V, Bremner JD. Traumatic stress is heartbreaking. Biol Psychiatry. 2013;74(11):790–2.

Interstitial Pulmonary Disease After Exposure at the World Trade Center Disaster Site

Jaime Szeinuk

Introduction

Exposure to the airborne toxins that resulted from the attack to and subsequent collapse of the World Trade Center (WTC) has been reported to result in development of new-onset and persistent airway disease. This has been well documented by surveillance and clinical and epidemiological data [1–8].

In addition, several case reports and case series in the medical literature document the development of interstitial lung disease (ILD) [9–15] and distal airway disease with evidence of some involvement of the interstitial structures [3, 16] following exposures at the WTC disaster site. To the author's knowledge, no systematic epidemiological review of the incidence or prevalence of ILD in WTC-exposed individuals has been published up to date. This chapter will review the literature that suggests that ILD is likely to occur after exposure at the WTC disaster site. The chapter first discusses issues related to the nature of the WTC dust and which of its components have been causally linked to the development of ILD, subsequently analyzes exposure considerations based on the reported experience with WTC-related ILD conditions, and, finally, reviews the inflammatory response and clinicopathological evidence of WTC-related ILD conditions.

J. Szeinuk
Occupational and Environmental Medicine of Long Island, New Hyde Park, NY 11040, USA

Department of Occupational Medicine, Epidemiology and Prevention, Hofstra Northwell School of Medicine, Hempstead, NY 11549, USA
e-mail: jszeinuk@northwell.edu

WTC Dust

The destruction of the WTC towers produced a plume of a complex mixture of chemical agents in different forms. The plume contained the combustion products of jet fuel from the two commercial aircraft that crashed into the towers and the heating, diesel oil, and fuel from the several thousand automobiles and transformers that were destroyed when the towers collapsed, in addition to soot, metals, volatile organic compounds, and hydrochloric acid from the destroyed structures. The plume also contained particulate matter from pulverized building materials such as cement, glass, asbestos, crystalline silica, metals, polycyclic aromatic hydrocarbons, polychlorinated biphenyls, polychlorinated furans, organochlorine pesticides, and dioxins [17]. Lioy et al. [18] and Offenberg et al. [19] have reported on the composition and characteristics of collected settled dust samples in the immediate vicinity of the WTC site. By weight, at least 96% of these samples were composed of particulates larger than 10 μm in mass median aerodynamic diameter (MMAD). Respirable particulates including coarse particulates (PM_{10}: particulates >2.5 μm and <10 μm MMAD) and fine particulates ($PM_{2.5}$: particulates <2.5 μm MMAD) were found at much lower proportions (<1 and 0.5–4%, respectively). However, settled dust may not accurately represent the relative proportions of airborne respirable particulates following the collapse of the towers. Small particulates may coalesce or agglomerate to form larger particulates, altering the relative proportions of fine and coarse particulates. Bulk dust samples collected from the vicinity of the WTC area were composed of both fibrous and nonfibrous materials. Fibrous compounds included chrysotile asbestos, glass fibers, and fibers from cotton, wood, and paper (cellulose). Nonfibrous components included gypsum, calcite, bassanite (calcium sulfate hemihydrate), and quartz [20]. Composition of dust collected from indoor locations adjacent to the WTC site was similar [18, 21, 22]. A total of 287 chemicals or compounds to which people who came in contact with the cloud of dust from the WTC collapse were exposed have been identified. Information on these chemicals is kept by the Contaminants of Potential Concern (COPC) Committee of the World Trade Center Indoor Air Task Force Working Group [17].

There were no air sampling devices operating close to the WTC site at the time of the attacks and collapse of the towers to characterize and quantify the constituents of the dust cloud and smoke plumes. As a consequence, the people's exposures to the specific agents and concentrations in the early moments after the disaster will never be known with certainty [17]. By one estimation, the ambient fine particle mass concentration was approximately 500 μg/m³ of air on September 12, 2001 [23], which far exceeds the current US EPA 24-h air quality standard of 65 μg/m³ of air [24].

Banauch et al. [25] have classified the chemical toxic components of WTC dust into four categories: (1) particulate matter (calcium carbonate and silica) and fibers (chrysotile asbestos, fibrous glass, gypsum); (2) organic pollutants, including polycyclic aromatic hydrocarbons, other hydrocarbons (naphthalene, fluorine, polychlorinated biphenyl, dibenzo-p-dioxins, and diphenyl ethers), benzene, and Freon; (3)

gases, such as carbon monoxide, hydrogen sulfide, combustion by-products from the fires that burned until mid-December 2001, and diesel exhaust fumes from the vehicle/machinery employed; and (4) heavy metals (calcium, iron, zinc, aluminum, antimony, titanium, and magnesium). Additionally, Wu et al. [15] have identified carbon nanotubes (CNT) in the lungs of WTC patients and in WTC dust samples.

Exposure Categorization

Attempts to categorize the exposure of individuals to the attacks and collapse of the towers and to the efforts of rescue, recovery, and restoration that continued until the end of December 2001, when the fires were finally extinguished, suggest that there were two significant initial time windows for a sufficient exposure that could have resulted in significant health consequences. The first one corresponds to the initial 5–6 h after the actual collapse of the towers, when the earliest release and distribution of the pulverized building materials and plume emissions caused by the jet fuel fires occurred. The second one occurred between September 11 and 14, 2001. During this time, fires were still burning, and the highest levels of re-suspendable particulate mass could be mobilized from surfaces. This period probably ended with the first post-September 11 rains, which may have decreased the intensity of the fires, washed away the settled re-suspendable materials, and thus reduced exposure to ambient background levels [23]. However, during the days that followed September 14, intermittent releases of high concentrations of gaseous substances and particulate matter into the local atmosphere within the Ground Zero area still occurred, caused by uncovered fires and the disturbance of settled dust by rescue workers during debris movement and removal [23]. Smoldering fires continued for some 4 months after the initial attack, during which WTC dust was released and aerosolized [26]. Rescue/recovery efforts finally concluded by the end of May 2002 [26].

Additionally, there was exposure in the indoor environment, in dwellings and offices, and in other commercial buildings in close proximity to the site. Given the facts that conditions of affected residences and buildings were not uniform and that people responded differently in their attitudes to confront such exposures, the estimate of this exposure is virtually impossible in terms of general characterization [23].

Assessment of the exposure during the disaster response has been carried out by a variety of means. Environmental air samples collected between September 18 and October 4, 2001, have been reported [27]. Personal air sample results collected from the breathing zones have been reported in truck drivers [28, 29] and emergency responders [30]. Biomonitoring has been carried out in firefighters [31, 32] and in National Guard and New York State personnel [33, 34]. Measured agents in the different published papers included asbestos, concrete, crystalline silica, carbon monoxide, diesel exhaust, chlorodifluoromethane, heavy metals (e.g., cadmium, mercury), hydrogen sulfide, inorganic acids, particulate matter (including PM_{10} and

$PM_{2.5}$), total dust, volatile organic compounds, perfluorochemicals, polychlorinated aromatic hydrocarbons (such as benzopyrene, hydroxypyrene, xylene), biphenyls (PCB), and dibenzodioxins and dibenzofurans. Overall, these studies show that the levels of measured agents generally remained within NIOSH Recommended Exposure Limits or Occupational Safety and Health Agency (OSHA) Permissible Exposure Limits, with exceptions including perfluorochemicals, polychlorinated aromatic hydrocarbons and dibenzofurans, lead and antimony, and cadmium and carbon monoxide, the two last ones associated mostly with the use of oxyacetylene torches. Measurements show an exposure/response relationship in that the earlier individuals were exposed to the plume or dust, the higher the concentrations found and also a gradient exposure ranging from measurements taken in close proximity to the pile to those taken at the perimeter.

Accounts of the exposure in the published case reports that describe ILD in WTC-exposed individuals show that the vast majority of the cases reported had sustained heavy exposure to the collapse, within the two window periods of heavy exposure as described by Lioy and Georgopoulos [23]. The firefighter who developed eosinophilic pneumonia [13] was present at the site on the day of the collapse of the towers and continued to work for periods of 16 h a day for 13 days. The patient who developed a granulomatous pneumonitis [14] was also exposed on the day of the collapse of the towers and then returned to the area for 1 day on September 14 and later on October 3, on a more regular basis. This patient worked at a building located one block away from the WTC. The NYC highway patrol officer who developed bronchiolitis obliterans [16] was exposed to the WTC dust on the day of the attacks and continued to work for periods of 16 h a day for 3 weeks when he first experienced symptoms. Patients included in the NYC firefighter series of "sarcoid-like" granulomas [11] were all present at the site within the initial 3 days after the collapse of the towers. Ten of the 26 reported patients had arrived in the morning of September 11, 2001, 14 arrived within the next 36 hours, and the last 2 arrived on day 3 after the attack. No specific information as to the duration of the exposure is reported in this article. Of the two cases that reported rheumatologic manifestations in WTC rescue workers with sarcoidosis [35], one was present during day 1 and continued working for some 3 months, while the second patient worked for some 6 months, starting on day 4 after September 11, 2001. The two cases with peripheral airway disease with extension to the parenchyma had worked at the disaster area for over 80 h before November 30, 2001 [3]. Of the 43 patients with sarcoidosis included in the WTC Health Registry report, 34 (79%) sustained their initial exposure within the first 4 days after the attacks. Three of the remainder nine had to evacuate their homes because of the presence of WTC dust. This study documented that working on the WTC debris pile was associated with diagnosis of sarcoidosis [12]. No "statistically significant trend" between level of exposure and diagnosis of sarcoid-like granulomatous disease was found in the series described by Crowley et al. [10]. Finally, only two of the six cases of local residents who underwent pulmonary biopsies and presented with an "interstitial" disease pattern were present in the initial dust cloud; however, no additional information on duration of exposure was provided [9].

Identification of WTC Dust in the Respiratory Tract

There are several reports on the characterization and composition of the WTC dust deposited in the airways or pulmonary tissue of individuals who were exposed and/or developed diseases as a consequence of their exposure.

Rom et al. [13] reported on bronchoalveolar lavage (BAL) analyses in a firefighter hospitalized with acute eosinophilic pneumonitis several weeks after WTC exposure. Significant quantities of fly ash, degraded fibrous glass, and asbestos fibers were found. BAL revealed 305 fibers per million alveolar macrophages. Types of fibers included chrysotile and amosite asbestos, chromium, and predominantly silica-containing fibers that were attributed to degraded fibrous glass. A variety of nonfibrous particles were identified, including fly ash, silica, metal particles, and various silicates. The fact that only uncoated asbestos fibers were found was interpreted as indicative of recent exposure since coated asbestos bodies are expected in more regular, chronic exposure.

A study of induced sputum samples from nonsmoking New York City firefighters exposed to WTC dust (NY-FF), some 10 months after the collapse of the WTC towers, was reported in 2004 [32]. The firefighters' exposure duration varied from 1 to 75 days. Induced sputum is a noninvasive alternative to study inhaled particle matter and the lung's inflammatory response to inhaled toxins and has yielded similar results to BAL in silica and hard metal workers and other patients with occupational lung diseases [36]. Induced sputum findings on NY-FF were compared to those in a control population of Israeli hospital workers free from respiratory disease and also with a group of Tel Aviv firefighters (TA-FF). The study showed that the NY-FF samples contained a higher percentage of particulates of size >2 and >5 μm than TA-FF, but no relationship between particle size and length of stay at the WTC area was found. Particles found in NY-FF were irregularly shaped as compared to the smaller, regularly shaped particles found in TA-FF. Chemical and mineralogical analyses of these particles revealed metal alloys and oxides consistent with the composition of WTC dust and different from that of non-WTC-exposed firefighters. These mineral particles were seen within the macrophages and epithelial cells of the NY-FF. Minerals detected included silica in three out of four samples and aluminum and magnesium silicates in one of the samples, in addition to metals found in the WTC building components, including titanium, iron, calcium, nickel, chromium, and zinc.

Wu et al. [15] described mineralogical findings in seven previously healthy responders who were exposed to WTC dust on either September 11 or 12, 2001, and developed severe respiratory impairment or unexplained radiologic findings. Tissue analyses showed large amounts of aluminum and magnesium silicates in an unusual sheet configuration in all those who had interstitial disease. Four of the seven patients with interstitial lung disease had single-walled CNT of various lengths. Chrysotile asbestos, calcium phosphate and calcium sulfate, and small shards of glass containing mostly silica and magnesium were identified in some cases as well.

More recently, Caplan-Shaw et al. [9] published on scanning electron microscopy of tissue blocks in five of twelve local workers, residents, and cleanup workers exposed to WTC dust who underwent surgical lung biopsy for suspected interstitial lung disease. All had presence of particles on light microscopy, but not an overwhelming number. Silica was detected in individual particles in four of the five patients. Aluminum silicates, titanium dioxide, and talc particles were also found. All cases had metals identified in the particles, including aluminum, steel, zirconium, chromium, copper, zinc, and tin.

Toxicological Effects in Laboratory Animals and Cultured Cells

Mice exposed to oropharyngeal aspiration of 100 μg (microgram) samples of WTC dust particles with a MMAD of less than 2.5 μm ($PM_{2.5}$) exhibited a slight increase in BAL neutrophils. In addition, this exposure caused significant airflow obstruction in response to methacholine challenge. Lower doses administered directly into the airways (32 and 10 μg) or nasal inhalation of 11 mg/m^3 WTC $PM_{2.5}$ for 5 h did not induce significant inflammation or airflow obstruction. These results suggest that there may be a threshold dose for respiratory effects of WTC $PM_{2.5}$ in healthy mice. Theoretical calculations indicate that the 100 μg dose in mice corresponds to inhalation of 425 μg/m^3 WTC $PM_{2.5}$ for 8 h by humans to achieve a comparable dose in the tracheobronchial region. Such exposures likely existed immediately after the collapse of the WTC towers, especially given the lack of sufficient respiratory protection in most rescue personnel. However, most individuals would not be expected to experience such exposures if they were not caught in the dust cloud immediately after the collapse of the towers [37].

Studies in cultured human alveolar macrophages and type II cells exposed to the $PM_{2.5}$ fraction of indoor and outdoor WTC collected settled dust showed dose-dependent increases in pro-inflammatory cytokines such as tumor necrosis factor alpha, interleukin (IL)-8, and IL-6 and in gamma-glutamyl transpeptidase (GGT), a membrane-bound enzyme that transfers extracellular precursors of the antioxidant glutathione into the cell cytoplasm where it protects against oxidative tissue damage. The coarse and very coarse fractions of WTC PM caused similar though generally lower responses in these cell types [38]. An additional study has shown that the mitogen-activated protein kinase signaling pathway is activated in a dose-dependent manner by WTC dusts, which could play an important role in the production of inflammatory cytokines [39].

Inflammatory Markers in Response to WTC Dust Exposure

Inflammatory markers have been reported in studies of induced sputum and BAL from patients who developed lung disease due to WTC exposure.

The BAL of the NYC firefighter who was hospitalized with acute eosinophilic pneumonitis several weeks after WTC exposure [13] had a significant inflammatory response with elevated number of cells recovered (730,000 compared to a normal of less than 250,000), 70% of which were eosinophils. The eosinophils were not degranulated. Lymphocyte subpopulations (B cells, NK cells, CD8+ cells, and CD4 T cells) were normal, but the alveolar CD4+ lymphocytes exhibited a highly stimulated surface phenotype. IL-5, an eosinophilic chemotactic factor, was elevated.

Inflammatory markers were studied on induced sputum from nonsmoking NY-FF some 10 months after the collapse of the WTC towers and compared with markers in induced sputum of TA-FF and an unexposed control population of hospital workers [32]. NY-FF and TA-FF had significantly more neutrophils, lymphocytes, and eosinophils and fewer macrophages than hospital workers, but differential cell counts were not different between NY-FF and TA-FF. Percentage of neutrophils and eosinophils significantly increased with longer exposure at the WTC area, thus suggesting a dose (exposure)-response (inflammation) relationship. Higher levels of matrix metalloproteinase-9 (MMP-9) were found in NY-FF as compared to TA-FF and to non-firefighters. MMP-9 plays an important role in neutrophil recruitment to the lungs. It is reliably and reproducibly detectable in induced sputum and has been shown to be elevated in workers exposed to hazardous dust. This elevation was interpreted as evidence for exposure-related immune activation in the lungs, which was persistent some 10 months after WTC dust exposure.

Interstitial Lung Disease Due to WTC Exposure: Clinicopathological Responses

Two main clinicopathological responses have been documented in case series of WTC-exposed individuals with ILD reported in the medical literature: a granulomatous response and a "diffuse pulmonary fibrosis"-type response. Other papers have identified single cases with different clinicopathological responses, some of which have been presented above.

Several studies have documented a granulomatous response to WTC exposure. An initial report described a non-sarcoid granulomatous pneumonitis in a WTC-exposed individual [14]. Lung biopsy of this patient demonstrated non-caseating granulomata with silica, silicate, and calcium oxalate particles. The patient was acutely ill and recovered with corticosteroid therapy. Izbicki et al. [11] reporting on surveillance data among NYC firefighters suggested an increased incidence after September 11, 2001, of "sarcoid-like" granulomatous pulmonary disease, in comparison with before that date. This study included 26 NYC firefighters with "sarcoid-like" granulomatous pulmonary disease. Inclusion into this study required pathology finding of non-caseating granulomas without evidence for foreign body reaction, malignancy, or fungal or mycobacterial infection. Nine patients presented with adenopathy only, and the remaining 17 had adenopathy and parenchymal disease. Only three of the cases had a total lung capacity and/or diffusion capacity below 80% of predicted, and extra-thoracic disease was present in 23% of the cases.

Half of the cases were reported within a year after September 11, 2001, and the remaining half over the following 4 years. Bowers et al. [35] reported two cases of WTC rescue workers who presented with extrapulmonary rheumatologic manifestations. The first patient initially presented with shortness of breath on exertion concomitantly with severe joint pain and swelling involving ankles and knees, as well as painful erythematous lesions on his legs consistent with erythema nodosum. The second patient presented with relapsing uveitis followed by swelling of his ankles, left knee, and left elbow. Both patients had hilar adenopathy identified on CT scans, with no reported parenchymal abnormalities. Crowley et al. [10] reported on their findings of sarcoid-like granulomatous pulmonary disease among a population of some 19,756 responders examined through the WTC Medical Monitoring and Treatment Program. Cases were identified by self-report, physician report, and ICD-9 codes and evaluated by three pulmonologists to include only "definite" cases. Thirty-eight patients were classified as "definite" cases of sarcoid-like granulomatous pulmonary disease, with a peak incidence in the year between September 11, 2003, and September 11, 2004. Incidence in black responders was nearly double that of white responders. Nineteen patients had lymphadenopathy only, and 15 had adenopathy and parenchymal disease, with the remaining having normal radiographs (3) or x-rays not available for review (1). Twelve of 26 with acceptable quality spirometry had a low forced vital capacity (FVC), and 14 had normal spirometry. Jordan et al. [12] reported on biopsy-proven sarcoidosis post-9/11 among some 46,322 individuals who are part of the NYS WTC Health Registry. Cases were defined as sarcoidosis if confirmed by demonstration of non-caseating granulomas and the absence of any known granulomagenic organism or particle on tissue biopsy performed after October 2001, as verified by the authors. Forty-three cases fulfilled inclusion criteria, out of 430 who initially reported having been diagnosed with sarcoidosis. Twenty-seven cases had lymphadenopathy only, seven had parenchymal abnormalities by CT (although not necessarily nodules) only, and four had both. The remaining cases were either normal (two) or had radiography not available. Extra-thoracic involvement was present in 44%. Cases were overall evenly diagnosed between 2002 and 2006, with much less proportion of cases diagnosed in 2007 and 2008. There is no mineralogical information reported on the tissue biopsies of these cases, except for the requirements of "non-evidence of foreign body reaction or particles in biopsy." Mineralogical information in granulomatous responses associated with WTC exposure has been reported in an analysis of patients from the World Trade Center Environmental Health Center who were diagnosed with sarcoidosis after their exposure to WTC dust. This abstract reported silica and aluminum silicates in a limited mineralogical analysis of lymph node and parenchymal biopsy specimens (Parsia et al., cited in [9]).

Two case series have reported a "diffuse pulmonary fibrosis"-like response to the WTC exposure. Wu et al. [15] reported seven patients who underwent pulmonary biopsy because of severe respiratory impairment or radiologic findings. Table 1 summarizes the findings of this case series. All the patients except for case 6 are

Table 1 Summary of cases with interstitial findings presented in the Wu et al. paper

Case no.	Clinical history	Pathology findings/ mineralogical findings	PFT findings	Chest CT scan findings
1	Shortness of breath, hoarseness, cough, wheezing, asthma, bronchitis, pneumonia	Interstitial pulmonary fibrosis with subpleural distribution, prominent mediastinal nodules. AS, MS, CNT	Severe restrictive, low DLco	Honeycombing, severe peripheral fibrosis, peribronchiolar Usual interstitial fibrosis (UIP) like fibrosis
2	Dyspnea, cough, throat irritation, wheezing	7 small nodules, prominent interstitial markings, bronchiectasis. CNT, AS, MS, no asbestos	Mild restrictive/ obstructive, O_2 desaturation on exercise	Bronchiolocentric interstitial fibrosis, multiple patterns: UIP. Nonspecific interstitial pneum onia (NSIP), hypersensitivity
3	Cough, dyspnea on exertion	Subpleural interstitial linear and ground glass changes, enlarged lymph nodes. Chrysotile, AS, MS, CNT	Severe restriction, low DLco	Peribronchiolar fibrosis, NSIP type, extensive lymphocytic infiltrates and bronchiolitis
4	Dry cough, sore throat, hoarseness, wheezing, GERD, diarrhea	Mosaic lung. CNT, AS, MS, calcium sulfate, chrysotile	Moderate restriction	Bronchiolitis, mild peribronchiolar fibrosis
5	Shortness of breath on effort, chest pain, wheezing	Peripheral changes suggestive of UIP, lymph nodes mildly enlarged. AS, MS, chrysotile	Mild restriction, low DLco	Focal areas of fibrosis with fibroblastic foci small granulomas, non-necrotizing, peribronchiolar lesions. Airways: mucopurulent
6	Dry cough, wheezing	Marked mosaic pattern. No mineral detected	Normal spirometry and DLco	Small airway disease, respiratory bronchiolitis, peribronchial metaplasia, lung parenchyma unremarkable
7	Dyspnea on exertion, cough, wheezing, chest tightness	Multiple nodules, some calcified, peribronchial interstitial disease. MS, chrysotile	Minimal restriction, positive bronchodilator response	Granulomas non-necrotizing epithelioid

nonsmokers. All the patients with interstitial disease had large amounts of aluminum silicates (AS) and magnesium silicates (MS), in what was described as an "unusual platy configuration." Both the configuration of the silicates and the excessive amount of silicates were not found in a comparison group of construction workers heavily exposed to asbestos in the course of their work. Additionally, the lung specimens of three of the patients with interstitial fibrosis contained CNT that were virtually identical to those identified in samples of settled WTC dust. CNT were not found in lung samples of a control population of construction workers. Small airway disease was present in almost all cases with different degrees of severity. Interstitial disease was present in four cases, characterized by a generally bronchiolocentric pattern of interstitial inflammation and fibrosis of variable degree of severity.

Caplan-Shaw et al. [9] report on 12 patients who underwent surgical lung biopsy for suspected interstitial lung disease or abnormal pulmonary function tests. Table 2 summarizes the findings of this case series. The authors divided their patients into

Table 2 Summary of cases with interstitial disease presented in the Caplan-Shaw paper

Case no.	Pathology findings/ mineralogical findings (MF)	PFT findings	Chest CT scan findings
Interstitial disease on HRCT			
1	Moderate fibrosis, small airway fibrosis. MF not available	Restrictive, low DLco	Mild reticulation and bronchiectasis, mostly subpleural in lower lobes
2	Severe fibrosis, honeycombing, small airway fibrosis. AS, silica, titanium, talc	Restrictive/obstructive, markedly low DLco	Severe reticulation, moderate bronchiectasis, upper and lower lobes, diffuse
3	Moderate fibrosis, cellular infiltrates, granuloma, small airway fibrosis. AS, silica, titanium, talc	Unable to perform	Moderate reticulation, severe bronchiectasis, moderate ground glass opacity and mosaic attenuation, lower lobe, diffuse
4	Granuloma, organizing pneumonia, no fibrosis and no small airway fibrosis. MF not available	Normal, DLco not available	Mild reticulation, mild mosaic attenuation, lower lob, subpleural
5	Severe fibrosis, honeycombing, organizing pneumonia, small airway fibrosis. MF not available	Restrictive, severely decreased DLco	Marked reticulation and bronchiectasis, honeycombing, all lobes, diffuse
6	Severe fibrosis, honeycombing, small airway fibrosis. MF not available	Restrictive, mildly decreased DLco	Moderate reticulation, mild bronchiectasis, all lobes, subpleural

Table 2 (continued)

Case no.	Pathology findings/ mineralogical findings (MF)	PFT findings	Chest CT scan findings
No interstitial findings on HRCT			
7	Small airway fibrosis. MF not available	Restrictive, moderately reduced DLco	Mild mosaic attenuation, upper and lower lobes, air trapping
8	Granuloma, small airway fibrosis. AS, silica, titanium, talc	Restrictive/obstructive, DLco not available	Diffuse bronchial wall thickening, lower lobe
9	Moderate fibrosis, granuloma, small airway fibrosis. AS, titanium, talc, no silica	Restrictive, moderately reduced DLco	Marked ground glass and mosaic attenuation, diffuse bronchial wall thickening and air trapping
10	Granuloma, small airway fibrosis. MF not available	Restrictive/obstructive, mildly reduced DLco	Moderate mosaic attenuation, diffuse bronchial wall thickening and air trapping
11	Moderate fibrosis, no small airway fibrosis. AS, silica, titanium, talc	Restrictive, mildly reduced DLco	Minimal air trapping
12	Emphysema	Restrictive, mildly reduced DLco	None

two groups: those with predominant "interstitial" disease on HRCT and those who had abnormal physiology and HRCT abnormalities but not "interstitial" findings. Authors state that when identified, granulomas were scant and poorly formed. Pathological analysis identified emphysematous changes in all but one patient (case 10) and mild and patchy cellular infiltrates in all but one patient (case 12). All cases had opaque particles consistent with combustion products and birefringent particles containing inorganic compounds, including silica and aluminum silicates, as well as titanium dioxide and other metals identified within macrophages. Their analysis was not able to detect nanotubes or asbestos fibers.

Constrictive bronchiolitis has been documented histologically in three WTC-exposed workers [3, 16] and suggested radiologically in several others [16]. While this entity is excluded from the histological definition of ILD, one case reported in a WTC-exposed worker [16] demonstrated chronic bronchiolitis, focal obliterative bronchiolitis, and rare non-necrotizing granulomas in the parenchyma on open lung biopsy. Histological findings in a second case included focal and mild interstitial fibrosis with lymphocyte aggregates but without fibroblastic foci or honeycombing [3]. In a third case, end-expiratory air trapping was documented together with peri-bronchiolar fibrosis in association with severe restriction, reduced diffusion capacity, and radiologic and histological interstitial pulmonary fibrotic changes [3]. Thus, in these three cases of primarily distal airway disease, there is histopathological evidence suggesting some degree of extension of the inflammatory process more distally into the interstitial space.

Discussion

The development of environmentally induced pulmonary fibrosis can be conceptualized as starting with the inhalation of the causative agent. Physical characteristics of the inhaled toxin (e.g., dimensions, solubility), chemical composition, dose, and lung clearance mechanisms (including anatomic and physiologic characteristics of the airways, presence of disease, and minute ventilation) all contribute to the delivery of the agent to the alveolar spaces and affect the distribution, uptake and retention of the toxin at the lung parenchyma, and its potential to cause lung injury [40]. Analyses of WTC dust as reviewed above demonstrated that some percentage of the dust was composed of particles small enough to penetrate deep into the pulmonary system and to reach distal airways and alveoli [18, 19, 41]. The presence and retention of such particles has been confirmed in studies of induced sputum and BAL in WTC-exposed firefighters [13, 32] and in pathology studies of lung tissue from individuals involved in rescue and recovery work [14, 15] as well as from community residents [9]. The two main series and the limited review on granulomatous responses that have described mineralogy composition of the pathology samples of the lungs from WTC-exposed individuals consistently report the presence of silica and aluminum and magnesium silicates, in addition to other mineral findings [9, 15]. It appears so far that these silicates may be the primary agents responsible for the generation of the inflammatory response that results in ILD in WTC-exposed patients.

Following their retention in the pulmonary tissue, and either by their chemical and/or physical characteristics, the inhaled toxins injure the alveolar epithelial cell, dysregulating normal homeostatic wound healing and repair pathways mediated by epithelial mesenchymal interaction, resulting in fibroblast activation and proliferation and continued pathologic production of a provisional matrix primarily of interstitial collagens [42]. Variations in the pattern of immunologic response, probably genetically determined, play a major role on the individual's response to the injury and the final development of persistent damage and disease [40]. As previously reviewed herein, animal, in vitro studies, and case reports all suggest that WTC dust is capable of inducing a pulmonary inflammatory response. Animal models [37] and cell culture models [38] have shown the ability of the dust to induce production of inflammatory mediators. Studies of induced sputum and of BAL in firefighters and in patients who developed disease as a result of their exposure confirm the presence of elevated levels of matrix metalloproteinases and interleukins and alteration in the number and the immunologic properties of pulmonary parenchymal inflammatory cells [13, 32]. Two main inflammatory responses have been described in series that document findings of ILD in individuals exposed to WTC fumes: a granulomatous response [10–12] and a patchy interstitial fibrosis in a predominant bronchiolocentric pattern [9, 15].

In most of the cases in which a clear environmental cause for ILD can be identified, clinical history usually reveals exposure to the toxin for long periods of time before development of symptoms [43–45] or for shorter periods of time (months) if the exposure was unusually heavy [26, 46, 47]. In the case of drug-induced lung disease, for example, fibrotic lung diseases develop after months to years of using the medication and sometimes even years after it has been stopped, except for acute, idiosyncratic reactions [48]. Similarly, in cases of hypersensitivity pneumonitis, exposure to the sensitizing agent usually occurred over a long period of time [49]. Almost all of the pneumoconioses present after long latency periods. These points illustrate the need to accrue and retain significant amounts of toxins in the lung parenchyma in order to trigger clinical disease and to allow for sufficient latency time for symptoms and clinical findings to manifest. The one common denominator in the vast majority of the cases of post-WTC exposure ILD summarized above is the fact that the affected patients were exposed during the period when the environmental concentration of WTC dust was at its highest, i.e., during the day of the attacks and/or up to 3 days after the collapse of the towers, thus allowing for a sufficient dose of inhaled WTC dust to generate a disease response. The one unusual issue in WTC-DPLD is the relative short latency between exposure and disease. Some of the reported cases of ILD related to exposure to WTC dust have been diagnosed within a short latency period after exposure, while others have been diagnosed several years after the attacks.

An additional unusual feature when comparing WTC-DPLD to other more "traditional" environmentally induced ILD is the lack of a common histopathological pattern. As stated in this review, the current literature has identified two major clinicopathological responses: a granulomatous inflammation and a more diffuse, interstitial-type response with a bronchiolocentric pattern, which we have termed "diffuse pulmonary fibrosis"-like in this chapter. Whereas the studies reported in the articles describing a granulomatous response have significant methodological differences, including recruitment, surveillance, and case ascertainment methods, and are all subject to reporting biases, the fact that this finding has been reported in three different populations (although with some overlap in between) gives some consistency to this finding. Similarly, the two case series that described a more diffuse, "diffuse pulmonary fibrosis"-like response to exposure to WTC dust present some similarities: CT images showed findings consistent with interstitial lung disease, and pathology demonstrated histologic patterns of patchy interstitial fibrosis, often in a bronchiolocentric pattern, with bronchiolitis and peribronchiolar fibrosis, and intracellular particles within collections of macrophages. Again, although the two studies had significant differences as to recruitment and surveillance of cases, the fact that similar clinicopathological responses have been reported in these two different populations gives some consistency to this finding as well.

In summary, at present the most frequently reported pulmonary consequence related to WTC exposure is airway disease. However, granulomatous responses, interstitial-like pulmonary disease, eosinophilic pneumonitis, and bronchiolitis obliterans with elements of extension into the parenchyma have all been reported. Most of these cases were exposed at the WTC site during the first few hours and days after the attack and the collapse of the towers, when the concentrations of inhalable toxicants are presumed to have been highest. Pathology and mineralogy studies have identified particles and toxicants within the macrophages at the distal airway/alveolar level. The presence of aluminum and magnesium silicates appears to be a common denominator in many of these cases. The variability in the reported pathological descriptions remains a challenge.

In conclusion, published reports so far suggest the possibility of development of an inflammatory response to WTC dust with clinicopathological consequences in the pulmonary tissue manifesting as ILD. Ongoing surveillance and follow-up of the cohort of exposed individuals are warranted, especially to allow for a longer latency period for these diseases to occur and to assess the additional potential for cumulative dose over time on the development of ILD.

References

1. Banauch GI, Alleyne D, Sanchez R, et al. Persistent hyper reactivity and reactive airway dysfunction in firefighters at the World Trade Center. Am J Respir Crit Care Med. 2003;168:54–62.
2. Buyantseva LV, Tulchinsky M, Kapalka GMP, et al. Evolution of lower respiratory symptoms in New York police officers after 9/11: a prospective longitudinal study. J Occup Environ Med. 2007;49:310–7.
3. de la Hoz RE, Shohet MR, Chasan R, et al. Occupational toxicant inhalation injury: the World Trade Center experience. Int Arch Occup Environ Health. 2008;81:479–85.
4. Feldman DM, Baron SL, Bernard BP, et al. Symptoms, respiratory use, and pulmonary function changes among New York City firefighters responding to the World Trade Center Disaster. Chest. 2004;125:1256–64.
5. Herbert R, Moline J, Skloot G, et al. The World Trade Center Disaster and the health of workers: five-year assessment of a unique medial screening program. Environ Health Perspect. 2006;114:1853–8.
6. Mendelson DS, Roggeveen M, Levin SM, et al. Air trapping detected on end-expiratory high resolution CT in symptomatic World Trade Center rescue and recovery workers. J Occup Environ Med. 2007;49:840–5.
7. Prezant DJ, Weiden M, Banauch GI, et al. Cough and bronchial responsiveness in firefighters at the World Trade Center Site. N Eng J Med. 2002;347:806–15.
8. Wheeler K, McKelvey W, Thorpe L, et al. Asthma diagnosed after September 11, 2001 among rescue and recovery workers: findings from the World Trade Center Health Registry. Environ Health Perspect. 2007;115:1584–90.
9. Caplan-Shaw CE, Yee H, Rogers L, Abraham JL, Parsia SS, Paidich DP, Borczuk A, Moreira A, Shiau M, Ko JP, Brusca-Augello G, Berger KI, Glodring RM, Reibman J. Lung pathologic findings in a local residential and working community exposed to World Trade Center dust, gas and fumes. J Occup Environ Med. 2011;53:981–1.
10. Crowley LE, Herbert R, Moline JM, Wallenstein S, Shukla G, Schechter C, Skloot GS, Udasin I, Luft BJ, Harrison D, Shapiro M, Wong K, Sacks HS, Landigran PJ, Teirstein AS. "Sarcoid like" granulomatous pulmonary disease in World Trade Center Disaster responders. Am J Ind Med. 2011;54:175–84.

11. Izbicki G, Chavko R, Banauch GI, et al. World Trade Center "sarcoid-like" granulomatous pulmonary disease in New York City Fire Department rescue workers. Chest. 2007;131:1414–23.
12. Jordan HT, Stellman SD, Prezant D, Teirstein A, Osahan SS, Cone JE. Sarcoidosis diagnosed after September 11, 2001, among adults exposed to the World Trade Center disaster. J Occup Environ Med. 2011;53:966–74.
13. Rom WN, Weiden M, Garcia R, et al. Acute eosinophilic pneumonia in a New York City firefighter exposed to WTC dust. Am J Respir Crit Care Med. 2002;166:797–800.
14. Safirstein BH, Klukowicz A, Miller R, Teirstein A. Granulomatous pneumonitis following exposure to the World Trade Center collapse. Chest. 2003;123:301–4.
15. Wu M, Gordon RE, Herbert R, Padilla M, Moline J, Mendelson D, Litle V, Travis WD, Gil J. Case report: lung disease in World Trade Center responders exposed to dust and smoke: carbon nanotubes found in lungs of World Trade Center patients and dust samples. Environ Health Perspect. 2010;118:499–504.
16. Mann JM, Sha KK, Kline G, Breuer F-U, Miller A. World Trade Center dyspnea: bronchiolitis obliterans with functional improvement: a case report. Am J Ind Med. 2005;48:225–9.
17. National Institute for Occupational Safety and Health. First periodic review of scientific and medical evidence related to cancer for the World Trade Center Health Program. Department of Health and Human Services, NIOS Publication Number 2011-197, 2011.
18. Lioy PJ, Weisel CP, Mililerette JR, et al. Characterization of the dust/smoke aerosol that settled east of the World Trade Center in lower Manhattan after the collapse of the WTC 11 September 2001. Environ Health Perspect. 2002;110:703–14.
19. Offenberg JH, Eisenreich SJ, Chen LC, et al. Persistent organic pollutants in the dust that settled across lower Manhattan after September 11, 2001. Environ Sci Technol. 2003;37:502–8.
20. McGee JK, Chen LC, Cohen MD, et al. Chemical analysis of World Trade Center fine particulate matter for use in toxicological assessment. Environ Health Perspect. 2003;111:972–80.
21. Tang KM, Nace CG, Lynes CL, et al. Characterization of background concentrations in Upper Manhattan, New York apartments for select contaminants identified in World Trade Center Dust. Environ Sci Technol. 2004;38:6482–90.
22. Yiin LM, Millerette JR, Vette A. Comparisons of the dust/smoke particulate that settled inside the surrounding buildings and outside on the streets of southern New York City after the collapse of the World Trade Center, September 11, 2001. J Air Waste Manag Assoc. 2004;54:515–28.
23. Lioy PJ, Georgopoulos P. The anatomy of the exposures that occurred around the World Trade Center site, 9/11 and beyond. Ann NY Acad Sci. 2006;1076:54–79.
24. Johnson PRS, Graham JJ. Fine particulate matter National Ambient Air Quality Standards: public health impact on populations in the Northeastern United States. Environ Health Perspect. 2005;113:1140–7.
25. Banauch GI, Dhala A, Prezant DJ. Pulmonary disease in rescue workers at the World Trade Center site. Curr Opin Pulm Med. 2005;11:160–8.
26. Guidotti TL, Prezant D, de la Hoz R, Miller A. The evolving spectrum of pulmonary disease in responders to the World Trade Center tragedy. Am J Ind Med. 2011;54:649–60.
27. Centers for Disease Control. Occupational exposures to air contaminants at the World Trade Center disaster site – New York, September – October, 2001. MMWR. 2002;51:453–6.
28. Breysse PN, Williams DL, Herbstman JB, Symons JM, Chillrud SN, Ross J, Henshaw S, Rees W, Watson M, Geyh AS. Asbestos exposures to truck drivers during World Trade Center cleanup operations. J Occup Environ Hyg. 2005;2:400–5.
29. Geyh AS, Chillrud S, Williams DL, Herbstman J, Symons JM, Rees K, Ross J, Kim SR, Lim HJ, Turping B, Breysse P. Assessing truck driver exposure at the World Trade Center Disaster site: personal and area monitoring for particulate matter and volatile organic compounds during October 2001 and April 2002. J Occup Environ Hyg. 2005;2:179–93.
30. Wallingford KM, Snyder EM. Occupational exposure during the World Trade Center disaster response. Toxicol Ind Health. 2001;17:247–53.

31. Edelman P, Osterloh J, Pirkle J, Caudill SP, Grainger J, Jones R, Blount B, Calafat A, Turner W, Feldman D, Baron S, Bernard B, Lushniak BD, Kelly K, Prezant D. Biomonitoring of chemical exposure among New York City firefighters responding to the World Trade Center Fire and collapse. Environ Health Perspect. 2003;111:1906–11.
32. Fireman EM, Lerman Y, Ganor E, et al. Induced sputum assessment in New York City firefighters exposed to World Trade Center dust. Environ Health Perspect. 2004;112:1564–9.
33. Horii Y, Jiang Q, Hanari N, Lam PK, Yamashita N, Jansing R, Aldous KM, Mauer MP, Eadon GA, Kannan K. Polychlorinated dibenzo-p-dioxins, dibenzofurans, biphenyls, and naphtalenes in plasma of workers deployed at the World Trade Center after the collapse. Enrivon Sci Technol. 2010;44:5188–94.
34. Tao L, Kannan K, Aldous KM, Mauer MP, Eadon GA. Biomonitoring of perfluorochemicals in plasma on New York State personnel responding to the World Trade Center disaster. Environ Sci Technol. 2008;42:3472–8.
35. Bowers B, Hasni S, Gruber BL. Sarcoidosis in World Trade Center rescue workers presenting with rheumatologic manifestations. J Clin Rheumatol. 2010;16:26–7.
36. Fireman E, Greif J, Schwartz Y, et al. Assessment of hazardous exposure by BAL and induced sputum. Chest. 1999;115:1720–8.
37. Gavett SH, Haykal-Coates N, Highfill JW, et al. World Trade Center fine particulate matter causes respiratory tract hyper responsiveness in mice. Environ Health Perspect. 2003;11:981–91.
38. Payne JP, Kemp SJ, Dear W, et al. Effects of airborne World Trade Center dust on cytokine release by primary human lung cells in vitro. J Occup Environ Med. 2004;46:420–7.
39. Wang S, Prophete C, Soukup JM, Chen LC, Costa M, Ghio A, Qu QS, Cohen MD, Chen HG. Roles of MAPK pathway activation during cytokine induction in BEAS-2B cells exposed to fine World Trade Center dust. J Immunotoxicol. 2010;7:298–307.
40. Taskar VS, Coultas DB. Is idiopathic pulmonary fibrosis an environmental disease? Proc Am Thorac Soc. 2006;3:293–8.
41. Gavett SH. Physical characteristics and health effects of aerosols from collapsed buildings. J Aerosol Med. 2006;19:84–91.
42. Nair GB, Matela A, Kurbanov D, Raghu G. Newer developments in idiopathic pulmonary fibrosis in the era of anti-fibrotic medications. Exp Rev Resp Med. 2016;10:699–711. doi:10.1080/174/6348.2016.1177461. Accessed 19 May 2016
43. American Thoracic Society. Diagnosis and initial management of nonmalignant diseases related to asbestos. Am J Respir Crit Care Med. 2004;170:691–715.
44. American Thoracic Society. Adverse effects of crystalline silica exposure. Am J Respir Crit Care Med. 1997;155:761–5.
45. Mossman BT, Churg A. Mechanisms in the pathogenesis of asbestosis and silicosis. Am J Respir Crit Care Med. 1998;157:1666–80.
46. Ehlrich R, Lilis R, Chan E, Nicholson WJ, Selikoff IJ. Long term radiological effects of short term exposure to amosite asbestos among factory workers. Br J Ind Med. 1992;49:268–75.
47. Mossman BT, Ehrlich R, Lilis R, et al. Long-term radiological effects of short-term exposure to amosite asbestos among factory workers. Br J Ind Med. 1992;49:268–75.
48. Camus P, Fanton A, Bonniaud P, et al. Interstitial lung disease induced by drugs and radiation. Respiration. 2004;71:301–26.
49. Churg A, Muller NL, Flint J, Wright JL. Chronic hypersensitivity pneumonitis. Am J Surg Pathol. 2006;30:201–8.

Persistent Lower Respiratory Symptoms in the World Trade Center (WTC) Survivor Program, a Treatment Program for Community Members

Caralee Caplan-Shaw and Joan Reibman

Introduction: Populations at Risk for Health Effects

On September 11, 2001, Southern Manhattan was filled with the hundreds of thousands of people who visited, worked, lived, and studied in the financial and residential hub of New York City. In addition to the responders (firefighters, police, and volunteer construction and utility workers) who rushed to the site, approximately 300,000 of these community members were at risk for exposure after the WTC disaster. This group included more than 250,000 local workers, 8000 grade school students, 45,000 college students, and more than 60,000 residents living south of Canal Street [1]. On the day of the disaster, some were hit with falling debris when the planes crashed through the buildings, others were caught in the massive dust cloud produced by the collapse of the towers, and still others wandered for hours in the dust before finding their way out of the area [2].

The ensuing chaos brought on by the unprecedented disaster resulted in delays of assessment of potential health risks. Reassured by claims from the US Environmental Protection Agency (EPA) that "their air is safe to breathe," [3] huge numbers of area residents never left the area, and many resident evacuees and local workers returned to their homes and offices within a week after the event [2]). Since the area was not declared a toxic waste site, cleanup was unregulated, left to individual owners and tenants of dust-filled buildings in Southern Manhattan and parts of Brooklyn. Thus, workers and residents returned to indoor spaces whose interiors and ventilation systems were cleaned inconsistently or not at all, resulting in exposure of these individuals to resuspended dust and persistent odors from fires that burned for months [4, 5]. Although the New York City Department

C. Caplan-Shaw, M.D. (✉) • J. Reibman, M.D.
Division of Pulmonary and Critical Care Medicine, Department of Medicine,
Bellevue Hospital Center/NYU School of Medicine, New York, NY 10016, USA
e-mail: caralee.caplan-shaw@nyumc.org

© Springer International Publishing AG 2018   47
A.M. Szema (ed.), *World Trade Center Pulmonary Diseases
and Multi-Organ System Manifestations*, DOI 10.1007/978-3-319-59372-2_4

of Health and Mental Hygiene distributed leaflets with recommended cleaning techniques, most residents were unaware of them and proceeded to clean their apartments without personal protective equipment of any kind and in ways that were likely to have increased potential for dust inhalation [4, 6]. Cleanup workers hired by private companies similarly received little guidance on safe cleaning methods, and many were unofficially discouraged from using masks so as not to frighten their clients.

Toxicology and Health Effects in Responder Populations

Despite initial difficulties due to restricted access to the site and destruction of all local preexisting ambient air monitors, toxicologic studies of WTC dust and fumes accumulated over time. Preliminary information was presented at a symposium at Pace University in October 2001 [7] when the extreme alkalinity of the dust was revealed. Exposures were complex due to the massive amounts of pulverized materials (over 1.2 million tons), the chemical transformations occurring at high temperatures, resuspension of particles during rescue and recovery and cleaning attempts, and continuous release of fumes from fires [8]. Analyses of dust samples performed by university-based Environmental Health Sciences Research Centers funded by the National Institutes of Environmental Health Sciences showed that settled dusts were a mixture of building debris and combustion products, consisting of concrete, gypsum, synthetic vitreous fibers, metals, radionuclides, ionic species, and asbestos [4, 5, 9]. Chemical analyses revealed that the dusts were highly alkaline and contained polycyclic aromatic hydrocarbons, polychlorinated biphenyls, and other hydrocarbons [10, 11]. The dust was also found to be unusually aerosolizable, resulting not only in heavy acute exposures on the day of the disaster but chronic exposures from resuspension of dusts in indoor and outdoor spaces [8, 9].

Labor organizations and unions representing police officers, construction workers, and utility workers as well as physicians from the Fire Department of New York City (FDNY) argued the need for health surveillance given the substantial risks. With advocacy from these entities, a federally funded screening program for first responders only was initiated in July 2002 [12–14]. The first reports of adverse health effects were reported in firefighters, including "WTC cough" new-onset persistent upper and lower respiratory and gastrointestinal symptoms and reductions in lung function [15, 16]. After a federal program for treatment of WTC-related health effects in responders was established in 2006, research confirmed the presence of sinusitis, asthma-like illnesses, interstitial lung diseases, sarcoidosis-like lung disease, and gastroesophageal reflux that began or were aggravated by 9/11 exposures as well as an excess incidence of cancer [8, 17–21]. Studies in responders also showed a high prevalence of mental health conditions, including post-traumatic stress disorder, depression, and anxiety [12, 22–24].

Evolution of a Survivor Program

Implementation of health surveillance and treatment programs for at-risk community members lagged way behind those of responders [2]. Without early national advocacy, formal representation, or a system in place to coordinate research coupled with a barely functional postal service in the aftermath of the disaster, efforts to study health effects in community populations were difficult, requiring extensive fieldwork [2]. Despite the challenges, over 2800 residents completed surveys in English, Spanish, Mandarin, and Cantonese as part of a research study funded by the US Centers for Disease Control and Prevention (CDC) and completed by New York University/Bellevue Hospital in partnership with the New York State Department of Health and a coalition of community groups within 2 years of 9/11. Providing the first evidence of health effects in a local community population, the residents' respiratory health study compared these local residents to a control group living in Northern Manhattan and documented a greater than threefold increase in new-onset persistent respiratory symptoms associated with unplanned medical visits and use of rescue inhaler medications [25, 26]. The presence of physical damage, dust, and odors in the home was related to new-onset respiratory symptoms, with the greatest risk observed in those with an increased frequency or duration of dust or odors in their homes, suggesting a dose-response [27].

In 2003, the New York City Department of Health and Mental Hygiene and the federal Agency for Toxic Substance and Disease Registry launched the WTC Health Registry (WTCHR), a $20 million joint research program to collect data on the physical and mental health issues in WTC-exposed responders and community members. The WTCHR began enrollment in 2003 and confirmed the presence of respiratory symptoms in survivors of collapsed or damaged buildings in addition to reporting dose-response associations [1, 18, 21, 28, 29]. Subsequent studies by the registry documented increased asthma rates in children [30–32].

In response to the perceived need for care of community members with WTC exposures, the asthma clinic of Bellevue Hospital, the flagship hospital of New York City's public health system, launched a small, unfunded community treatment program. The program expanded in 2005 from a clinic serving a few hundred to a program enrolling thousands with the help of funding from the American Red Cross Liberty Disaster Relief Fund. Thanks to advocacy from community organizations, an additional 5 years of funding was secured from the City of New York in 2006. In 2008, again in response to pressure from community organizations and local politicians, federal money was provided for the first time through a 3-year grant awarded by the National Institute for Occupational Safety and Health (NIOSH) for provision of medical and mental health treatment to community members with symptoms after 9/11 exposures [33].

In 2010, Congress passed the James Zadroga 9/11 Health and Compensation Act, which created a World Trade Center Health Program (WTCHP) with Centers of Excellence with expertise in screening, monitoring, and comprehensive treatment of WTC-related conditions for "responders" and "survivors" (community members). The clinical care is closely monitored, and treatment is provided only for conditions that are "certified" by a physician as having been caused, contributed to, or aggravated by confirmed WTC exposures. There was great political resistance to including community members in the bill: many assumed community members had insignificant exposures compared to responders and were not at risk, and most were concerned about the costs of ongoing treatment of such a large group of people. Through the concerted efforts of community groups, labor organizations, and local politicians, community members were eventually written into the bill, although with conditions and restrictions on coverage. Whereas "responders" undergo routine surveillance (monitoring) as well as treatment of certified conditions, "survivors" undergo monitoring only after diagnosis of a certified condition. "Responders" receive services at no cost; for "survivors," personal insurance is billed first, and the WTCHP is the secondary payor. As of August 2015, over 62,700 "responders" were enrolled for surveillance and over 24,000 for treatment of a certified condition; 8475 "survivors" were enrolled for treatment only [2].

The Survivor Program at Bellevue Hospital: The World Trade Center Environmental Health Center (WTC EHC)

The Bellevue Hospital World Trade Center Environmental Health Center (WTC EHC) is a multidisciplinary medical and mental health treatment program for symptomatic community members exposed to WTC dust, gas, or fumes. Individuals present to the clinic in response to information about the program distributed by community organizations and local news reports. Inclusion in the program is based on an initial telephone screen to document potential WTC exposure as a local worker, resident, cleanup worker, or passerby in Southern Manhattan on or in the months after September 11, 2001, and the presence of any physical symptom that occurred or was exacerbated after September 11, 2001 [33].

At an initial visit, patients respond to a multidimensional interviewer-administered questionnaire to obtain information on demographic characteristics and confirm and characterize WTC exposures as a local worker, resident, or cleanup worker, student, or passerby; symptoms, including severity and temporal relationship to September 11, 2001; and functional status. Questionnaires are translated into Spanish, Mandarin, Cantonese, and Polish using Bellevue Hospital Center's remote, real-time translation system. Severity of dyspnea is assessed using the modified Medical Research Council (MRC) dyspnea scale. All patients undergo a standardized medical evaluation, including a detailed medical and exposure history and physical examination, a mental health screen, blood tests, chest radiograph, and pulmonary function studies, including spirometry and impulse oscillometry (IOS). When chest radiography is abnormal or spirometry shows a reduced forced vital capacity, further evaluation with high-resolution inspiratory expiratory computerized tomography (CT) of the chest and complete pulmonary function testing with plethysmography and diffusing capacity of carbon monoxide (DL_{co}) are performed. Patients may also undergo cardiac evaluation with exercise stress testing and echocardiogram, as clinically indicated. The WTC EHC treatment protocol includes treatment of asthmalike symptoms based on guidelines for asthma management [33]. Patients are subsequently invited for monitoring visits every 18 months, during which questionnaires and standardized evaluation are repeated [34].

Summary of Findings in Survivors

Exposures and Demographics

In contrast to assessment of exposure in responder populations, in whom time of arrival to the site and hours spent on the pile could be quantified to define exposure intensity, exposures among community members were varied, complex, changed over time, and occurred in both indoor and outdoor spaces [8]. Thus, the WTC EHC has defined exposures among survivors by exposure category (local worker, area resident, or cleanup worker) and by self-report of having been caught in the dust cloud [33]. Characteristics of the population as a whole and by exposure category are summarized in Table 1. In the early years of the program, when a small number of rescue and recovery workers were still included, local workers formed the largest

Table 1 Characteristics of WTC EHC population ($N = 1898$)

Characteristic, N (%)	Total (N = 1898)	Local worker (N = 709)	Resident (N = 378)	Cleanup worker (N = 566)	Rescue and recovery (N = 200)
Gender					
Male	1005 (53)	322 (45)	194 (51)	313 (55)	156 (78)
Age, mean ± SD	48 ± 12	50 ± 11	52 ± 14	43 ± 10	47 ± 10
Race					
White	867 (46)	309 (44)	158 (42)	247 (44)	130 (65)
Black	318 (17)	227 (32)	28 (7)	25 (4)	28 (14)
Asian	217 (11)	59 (8)	146 (39)	3 (1)	7 (4)
Other	48 (2)	22 (3)	3 (1)	12 (2)	6 (3)
No answer	448 (24)	92 (13)	43 (11)	279 (49)	29 (14)
Ethnicity					
Hispanic	792 (42)	172 (24)	68 (18)	482 (85)	57 (29)
Income/year					
≤30 K	1178 (62)	293 (41)	270 (71)	499 (88)	90 (45)
Insurance					
Uninsured	746 (39)	133 (19)	154 (41)	383 (68)	62 (31)
Tobacco					
≥5 pack years	423 (23)	182 (26)	103 (28)	74 (13)	62 (32)
Dust cloud	749 (40)	413 (60)	151 (41)	115 (21)	67 (34)

Adapted from [33]

exposure group (37%), with area residents comprising 19%, cleanup workers 30%, and rescue and recovery workers 11% of the population. Approximately 40% of patients reported having been exposed to the dust cloud; most of those caught in the dust cloud were area residents and workers [33].

The WTC EHC patient population is racially diverse, with nearly half of the group and most of the cleanup workers self-reporting as Hispanic. In contrast to firefighter and responder populations, survivors include a large proportion of women (nearly half), with a mean age of 48 at enrollment and little variation in age among the exposure groups. The vast majority have minimal or no smoking history. Residents and cleanup workers tended to have low incomes and no health insurance [33].

Symptoms

Although enrollment in the WTC EHC requires report of any physical symptom without any restriction as to the type of symptom, reported symptoms are similar to those reported in occupationally exposed rescue and recovery workers and include lower respiratory symptoms (LRS), nasal and sinus congestion, and gastroesophageal reflux symptoms. The first description of the WTC EHC population explored characteristics of nearly 2000 patients enrolled 4–7 years after September 11, 2001. Symptoms were considered "new" if they developed after 9/11 and "persistent" if they occurred ≥2 times per week in the month preceding evaluation. New-onset persistent lower respiratory symptoms in survivors are summarized in Fig. 1. Dyspnea on exertion and cough were the most common LRS (67% and 46%, respectively); some reported wheeze (27%) and chest tightness (28%). Nearly half of the population (41%) reported a modified MRC score of 3 or more, consistent with

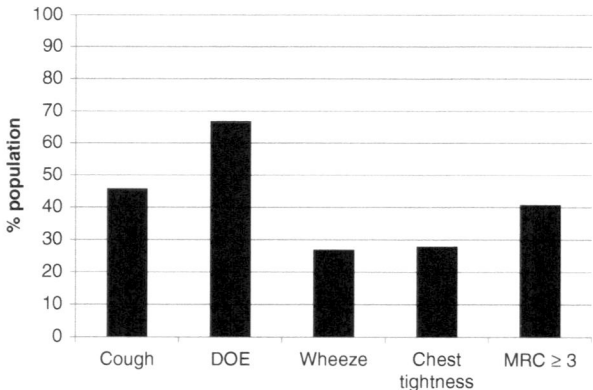

Fig. 1 Lower respiratory symptoms in the WTC EHC ($N = 1852$). Adapted from [33]. *$N = 1075$ for MRC ≥ 3

moderately to severely disabling dyspnea. Dust cloud exposure was significantly associated with new-onset persistent dyspnea on exertion and with moderately to severely disabling dyspnea in the area worker population [33].

Among both responder and survivor populations, an increased prevalence of persistent LRS has been associated with mental health symptoms, including posttraumatic stress disorder (PTSD), depression, and anxiety, even when adjusting for exposure intensity [28, 29, 35–38]. A study of nearly 2500 registry participants showed a dose-response relationship between the number of mental health conditions and poorer asthma control, with participants with three mental health conditions having five times the odds of very poor control compared to those without mental health issues [39]. Longitudinal data in responders demonstrated that PTSD increased the likelihood of development of LRS and decreased the rate of symptom remission [23]. Across all exposure types, LRS, especially in combination with PTSD, has been associated with reduced measures of quality of life [29]. A cross-sectional study of nearly 19,000 registry participants showed persistent LRS in nearly 15%, half of whom also had probable PTSD, depression, or anxiety and decreased quality of life 10 years after 9/11 [40].

Lung Function and Imaging

In the first description of WTC EHC patients, the vast majority (71%) had normal spirometry, and 90% had normal chest radiographs, consistent with findings in responder populations [33]. Spirometry was classified into normal and abnormal patterns using the lower limits of normal (LLN), defined as values below the lower fifth percentile, derived from the National Health and Nutrition Education Survey (NHANES) III population, as previously described [13, 41]. A low forced vital capacity (FVC) pattern was the most common abnormality and was associated with new-onset, persistent DOE [33]. The remaining patients with abnormal spirometry showed either an "obstructed" or combined "obstructed and low FVC" pattern. The distribution of the four spirometry patterns in the survivor population was consistent with other occupationally exposed populations [13] and with the spectrum of diseases that have been described in WTC-exposed responder populations, including reactive airway dysfunction, irritant-induced asthma, sarcoidosis, and interstitial lung diseases [16, 26, 42, 43]. These patterns have been studied in detail and suggest varied mechanisms of injury in WTC dust-exposed community members. The distribution of spirometry patterns in WTC EHC patients is provided in Table 2.

A normal spirometry pattern, seen in most survivors, can be seen in patients with no underlying lung disease but also in those with asthma or airway hyperresponsiveness. Alternatively, the possibility existed that exposed individuals with normal spirometry might have distal airway disease not reflected in spirometry [47, 48]. In a longitudinal analysis, FVC improved over time, suggesting reversible airway closure even in those with normal spirometry [44]. Additionally, in a subset of consecutive patients in the WTC EHC who underwent methacholine

Table 2 Spirometry patterns in WTC EHC patients with <5 pack-year tobacco history

Spirometry pattern	N (%)	Response to bronchodilator?	Longitudinal improvement?	Clinical associations
Normal	791 (71)		Yes	
Obstructed	67 (6)	Yes	Yes	Wheeze Elevated peripheral eosinophils
Low FVC	224 (20)	Minimal	Yes, but not to normal	New-onset persistent DOE Air trapping and bronchial wall thickening on CT
Obstructed and low FVC	28 (3)	Yes	Yes, greatest improvement but not to normal	Lowest spirometry parameters at baseline

Data from [33, 44–46]

challenge testing, nearly half showed airway hyperresponsiveness, a rate that is much higher than that reported in asymptomatic individuals [44, 49]. Airway hyperresponsiveness has been well described in firefighter and rescue and recovery populations [15, 16].

Although most patients with WTC exposures and LRS have been suggested to have asthma, an obstructed pattern is uncommon in the WTC EHC population as well as in other WTC-exposed groups [15, 16, 50]. In WTC EHC patients with an obstructed pattern, there was some improvement in spirometry parameters after administration of bronchodilator [33], and spirometry values improved over time, consistent with reversible airway disease [44]. Reinforcing the similarities to asthma in this group, an obstructive pattern was also associated with wheeze and elevated peripheral eosinophils [46]. Patients with an "obstructed and low FVC" pattern had the lowest spirometry values at baseline and showed improvement in both FVC and FEV_1 after administration of bronchodilator, suggesting airway disease with air trapping [33]. In a longitudinal analysis, this group showed the greatest improvement in FVC and FEV_1 over time [44].

Because the vast majority of symptomatic WTC-exposed individuals have normal spirometry, and because abnormalities of the distal airway may not be reflected in spirometry, multiple studies in a variety of WTC-exposed populations have used impulse oscillometry (IOS) to characterize the "quiet zone" of the lung. IOS measures include airway resistance (R_5, resistance at an oscillating frequency of 5 Hz), frequency dependence of resistance (R_{5-20}, the fall in resistance from 5 to 20 Hz), and heterogeneity of distal airway function (Ax, reactance area) [48, 51]. In a study of 174 WTC EHC patients with respiratory symptoms and normal spirometry, IOS values were elevated, and 37 of 43 were found to have frequency dependence of compliance by esophageal manometry, another measure of distal airway heterogeneity [51]. All parameters improved after administration of a bronchodilator. Since spirometry was normal in all subjects, the findings likely reflected at least partially reversible dysfunction in airways distal to those measured by spirometry. A nested case-control study of WTC Health Registry area residents and workers showed similar findings, with cases (individuals with LRS) substantially more likely than control subjects without LRS to have elevated airway resistance (R_5, 68% vs. 27%, $P < 0.0001$) and frequency dependence of resistance (R_{5-20}, 36% vs. 7%, $P < 0.0001$) [50]. These findings were reproduced in a larger study of 848 symptomatic WTC EHC patients compared to asymptomatic controls from WTC Registry, revealing higher IOS measures in symptomatic compared to asymptomatic subjects as well as an association between higher IOS values and increased severity and frequency of wheezing [52]. Finally, in a study of 166 symptomatic WTC EHC patients with normal spirometry undergoing bronchoprovocation with methacholine, 67 met spirometric criteria for bronchial hyperreactivity; however, an additional 24 patients had onset of LRS during bronchoprovocation coinciding with elevations in IOS values, suggesting the presence of isolated small airway reactivity as a mechanism for LRS [53].

The "low FVC" pattern, the most common abnormality found in both responder and survivor populations, can be seen in a variety of scenarios, including submaximal effort during lung function testing, parenchymal disease, obesity, or patchy peripheral air trapping [45]. In an effort to elucidate the etiology of the low FVC pattern in WTC EHC patients with lower respiratory symptoms, a retrospective physiologic study of 54 symptomatic subjects in the WTC EHC with reduced FVC and normal chest radiographs was undertaken [45]. Complete pulmonary function testing with plethysmography and DL_{co}, IOS measures, and inspiratory expiratory HRCT of the chest were analyzed. Lung function parameters suggested restriction due to air trapping; elevated IOS measures were found in 50 subjects, and imaging revealed bronchial wall thickening and/or air trapping in 40. In the 16 patients who underwent measurements of lung compliance, compliance was normal. In a study of 724 WTC EHC patients, elevated CRP levels (a marker of ongoing inflammation) were associated with the presence of LRS, elevated IOS parameters, and a low FVC pattern 6–11 years after 9/11, supporting the notion that ongoing inflammation may contribute to symptoms and distal airway dysfunction in survivors [54]. Taken together, these findings describe a distinct physiologic phenotype of restriction due to airway dysfunction. Studies in rescue and recovery workers [55] and firefighters [56] have similarly documented air trapping and bronchial wall thickening on CT scans associated with LRS and physiologic signs of airway dysfunction, including improvement in spirometry parameters after bronchodilator administration, elevated residual volume (a sign of air trapping), and airway hyperresponsiveness by methacholine challenge even in those with normal spirometry or a low FVC pattern.

Pathologic Findings

The ability of particulate matter to be inhaled and retained in the lung has been documented. Bronchoalveolar lavage fluid from a firefighter presenting with eosinophilic pneumonia contained large amosite asbestos fibers, fly ash particles, and degraded fibrous glass [57]. Induced sputum of New York City firefighters after 9/11 demonstrated inflammation and particles containing titanium [58]. Pathologic findings of bronchiolitis obliterans were found in a symptomatic responder [59]. In seven symptomatic WTC responders, histopathologic findings of small airway disease and bronchiolocentric parenchymal disease were identified in the presence of aluminum and magnesium sheet silicates, chrysotile asbestos, calcium phosphate, and calcium sulfate and, in some cases, carbon nanotubes [60].

Studies in survivors have shown similar findings. In a study of pathologic findings in survivors, lung function, high-resolution CT scans of the chest, and pathologic findings were reviewed in 12 patients who had undergone surgical lung biopsy for evaluation of suspected interstitial lung disease (ILD) or abnormal lung function [61]. While pulmonary function tests were predominantly restrictive, half of the group had radiologic findings consistent with ILD and half had normal or airway-related findings, including bronchial wall thickening or dilatation and air trapping. The predominant pathologic findings were interstitial fibrosis (mostly in those with ILD findings on CT), emphysematous changes, pulmonary arteriopathy, and small airway abnormalities, including bronchiolitis or small airway fibrosis associated with opaque and birefringent particles with macrophages. Analysis of tissue blocks by scanning electron microscopy with energy dispersive x-ray spectroscopy revealed silica, aluminum silicates, titanium dioxide, and talc, as well as metals (aluminum, steel, zirconium, chromium, copper, zinc, and tin) in concentrations not expected in a population without occupational exposure. Additionally, limited mineralogic analysis of WTC EHC patients with post-9/11 sarcoid also showed silica and aluminum silicates in lymph node and parenchymal biopsy specimens [62].

Longitudinal Assessment of LRS and Lung Function

In a longitudinal analysis of lung function in 946 patients in the WTC EHC, there was an overall improvement in spirometry parameters during an average 2.4-year follow-up period, with the degree of improvement varying by spirometry pattern at enrollment as described above as well as by exposure category and smoking status [44]. In contrast to the group as a whole, temporal improvement in lung function was not seen among heavy smokers. When stratified by WTC exposure category, longitudinal analysis indicated statistically significant improvement in lung function parameters among all exposure groups (local worker, resident, cleanup worker) with the exception of %FEV$_1$ in the cleanup group; local workers showed the least improvement over time. Additionally, longitudinal changes over time differed by spirometry pattern, as described above and summarized in Table 2.

A longitudinal assessment of nearly 800 WTC EHC patients showed minimal improvement in the proportion of patients with severe or mild LRS between initial and monitoring visits, with a majority of patients (63%) still meeting asthma guideline-based criteria for severe symptoms at monitoring (Fig. 2) [34]. Severe LRS at initial visit (present in 70%) was associated with dust cloud exposure, exposure as a local worker, elevated BMI, and the presence of mental health symptoms but not with spirometry. Among the 559 patients with severe LRS at initial visit, there were statistically significant improvements in functional status and frequency and severity of specific symptoms (cough, wheeze, chest tightness, and dyspnea) over time. The presence of PTSD or anxiety at initial visit was associated with persistence of severe LRS at monitoring; no other demographic or lung function parameters were distinguished between patients whose symptoms resolved or improved and those whose severe LRS persisted. As illustrated in Table 3, improvement in severe LRS was associated with improvements in distal airway function as measured by IOS, suggesting that LRS are not merely manifestations of mental health comorbidity but related to partially reversible abnormalities at the level of the distal airways.

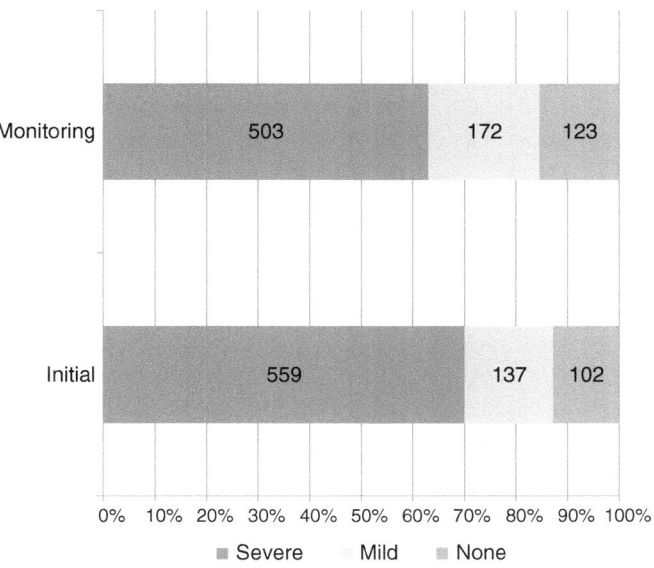

Fig. 2 Distribution of LRS severity at initial and monitoring visits ($n = 798$). Adapted from [34]

Table 3 Longitudinal change in spirometry and impulse oscillometry, by Symptom Trajectory, for the Severe LRS Group ($n = 559$)

	Resolved (47)	Improved (105)	Persistent (407)	P-value (K-W)	Trend test P-value
Spirometry delta (M1-V1) mean (SD)*					
FVC, % predicted	4.88 (2.77)	4.77 (2.55)	5.01 (2.51)	0.47	0.80
FEV$_1$, % predicted	3.66 (2.34)	3.84 (2.02)	3.84 (1.52)	0.11	0.11
FEV$_1$/FVC, %	0.91 (0.87)	0.88 (1.22)	1.04 (1.28)	0.12	0.08
Oscillometry delta δ = M1-V1, median (IQR)					
R$_{5-20}$, cm H$_2$O/L/s	−0.060 (0.47)	0.02 (0.65)	0.12 (0.83)		0.02

M1 monitoring visit, *V1* initial visit
Adapted from [34]

Conclusions and Future Questions for the Survivor Program

Taken together, studies in survivors show persistence of LRS many years after the WTC disaster associated with mental health symptoms and distal airway dysfunction. Although resolution or improvement in LRS is seen in a small proportion of patients associated with improvements in measures of distal airway function, the vast majority of survivors have persistent severe LRS and mental health symptoms impacting quality of life. Thanks to the Zadroga Act and ongoing federal funding for the survivor program, essential multidisciplinary care with concurrent treatment of medical and mental health issues will continue to be provided. Future studies in survivors are needed to consider the following questions:

What are the relative contributions of and relationships between mental health comorbidity and airway function, including distal airway function, in survivors with persistent LRS?
Does vocal cord dysfunction play a role in persistent LRS in survivors?
What are the pathophysiologic mechanisms of distal airway dysfunction in survivors with persistent LRS?
Can we improve treatment of persistent LRS in survivors with targeted therapies of the distal airway based on these pathophysiologic mechanisms?
What is the course of symptoms and lung function in survivors with persistent LRS due to interstitial lung disease?
Given the presence of pulmonary arteriopathy in lung tissue from survivors, does subclinical pulmonary vascular disease contribute to persistent LRS in survivors?

Funding Centers for Disease Control and Prevention (CDC)-National Institute for Occupational Services and Health (NIOSH) #200-2011-39413 Evaluation of Distal Airway Injury Following Exposure to World Trade Center Dust U01 OH011317 Small Airway COPD in the Survivor

Population U01OH010404 Uncontrolled Lower Respiratory Symptoms in WTC Survivor Population Clinical Center of Excellence: 1E11OH0030 (2008 – 2011) 200-2011-39391C (previous), 200-2017-93427 (current) Data Center: 200-2011-39379C (previous), 200-2017-93327 (current)

References

1. Brackbill RM, Thorpe LE, DiGrande L, Perrin M, Sapp JH II, Wu D, et al. Surveillance for world trade center disaster health effects among survivors of collapsed and damaged buildings. MMWR Surveill Summ. 2006;55(2):1–18.
2. Reibman J, Levy-Carrick N, Miles T, Flynn K, Hughes C, Crane M, et al. Destruction of the world trade center towers. Lessons learned from an environmental health disaster. Ann Am Thorac Soc. 2016;13(5):577–83.
3. Whitman CT. EPA press release. 2001.
4. Lioy PJ, Pellizzari E, Prezant D. The world trade center aftermath and its effects on health: understanding and learning through human-exposure science. Environ Sci Technol. 2006;40(22):6876–85.
5. Yiin LM, Millette JR, Vette A, et al. Comparisons of the dust/smoke particulate that settled inside the surrounding buildings and outside on the streets of southern new York City after the collapse of the world trade center, Sept 11, 2001. J Air Waste Manage Assoc. 2004;54(5):515–28.
6. New York City Department of Health, press release. Recommendations for people re-occupying commercial buildings and residents re-entering their homes. 17 Sept 2001.
7. Nadler J. U.S. congressman Jerrold Nadler white paper lower manhattan air quality. 2002.
8. Lippmann M, Cohen MD, Chen LC. Health effects of world trade center (WTC) dust: an unprecedented disaster's inadequate risk management. Crit Rev Toxicol. 2015;45(6):492–530.
9. Lioy PJ, Weisel CP, Millette JR, Eisenreich S, Vallero D, Offenberg J, et al. Characterization of the dust/smoke aerosol that settled east of the world trade center (WTC) in lower Manhattan after the collapse of the WTC 11 September 2001. Environ Health Perspect. 2002;110(7):703–14.
10. Butt CM, Diamond ML, Truong J, Ikonomou MG, Helm PA, Stern GA. Semivolatile organic compounds in window films from lower Manhattan after the September 11th world trade center attacks. Environ Sci Technol. 2004;38(13):3514–24.
11. Olson DA, Norris GA, Landis MS, Vette AF. Chemical characterization of ambient particulate matter near the world trade center: elemental carbon, organic carbon, and mass reconstruction. Environ Sci Technol. 2004;38(17):4465–73.
12. Crane MA, Levy-Carrick NC, Crowley L, Barnhart D, Dudas M, Onuoha U, et al. The response to September 11: a disaster case study. Ann Glob Health. 2014;80(4):320–31.
13. Herbert R, Moline J, Skloot G, Metzger K, Baron S, Luft B, et al. The world trade center disaster and the health of workers: five-year assessment of a unique medical screening program. Environ Health Perspect. 2006;114(12):1853–8.
14. Webber MP, Gustave J, Lee R, Niles JK, Kelly K, Cohen HW, et al. Trends in respiratory symptoms of firefighters exposed to the world trade center disaster: 2001–2005. Environ Health Perspect. 2009;117(6):975–80.
15. Feldman DM, Baron SL, Bernard BP, Lushniak BD, Banauch G, Arcentales N, et al. Symptoms, respirator use, and pulmonary function changes among new York City firefighters responding to the world trade center disaster. Chest. 2004;125(4):1256–64.
16. Prezant DJ, Weiden M, Banauch GI, McGuinness G, Rom WN, Aldrich TK, et al. Cough and bronchial responsiveness in firefighters at the world trade center site. N Engl J Med. 2002;347(11):806–15.

17. Banauch GI, Dhala A, Prezant DJ. Pulmonary disease in rescue workers at the world trade center site. Curr Opin Pulm Med. 2005;11(2):160–8.
18. Farfel M, DiGrande L, Brackbill R, Prann A, Cone J, Friedman S, et al. An overview of 9/11 experiences and respiratory and mental health conditions among world trade center health registry enrollees. J Urban Health. 2008;85(6):880–909.
19. Centers for Disease Control and Prevention. WTC health program at a glance. 2017. http://www.cdc.gov/wtc/ataglance.html
20. Guidotti TL, Prezant D, de la Hoz RE, Miller A. The evolving spectrum of pulmonary disease in responders to the world trade center tragedy. Am J Ind Med. 2011;54(9):649–60.
21. Maslow CB, Friedman SM, Pillai PS, Reibman J, Berger KI, Goldring R, et al. Chronic and acute exposures to the world trade center disaster and lower respiratory symptoms: area residents and workers. Am J Public Health. 2012;102(6):1186–94.
22. Bromet EJ, Hobbs MJ, Clouston SA, Gonzalez A, Kotov R, Luft BJ. DSM-IV post-traumatic stress disorder among world trade center responders 11-13 years after the disaster of 11 September 2001 (9/11). Psychol Med. 2016;46(4):771–83.
23. Kotov R, Bromet EJ, Schechter C, et al. Posttraumatic stress disorder and the risk of respiratory problems in world trade center responders: longitudinal test of a pathway. Psychosom Med. 2015;77(4):438–48.
24. Maslow CB, Caramanica K, Welch AE, Stellman SD, Brackbill RM, Farfel MR. Trajectories of scores on a screening instrument for PTSD among world trade center rescue, recovery, and clean-up workers. J Trauma Stress. 2015;28(3):198–205.
25. Lin S, Reibman J, Bowers JA, et al. Upper respiratory symptoms and other health effects among residents living near the world trade center site after September 11, 2001. Am J Epidemiol. 2005;162(6):499–507.
26. Reibman J, Lin S, Hwang SA, Gulati M, Bowers JA, Rogers L, et al. The world trade center residents' respiratory health study: new-onset respiratory symptoms and pulmonary function. Environ Health Perspect. 2005;113(4):406–11.
27. Lin S, Jones R, Reibman J, Bowers J, Fitzgerald EF, Hwang SA. Reported respiratory symptoms and adverse home conditions after 9/11 among residents living near the world trade center. J Asthma. 2007;44(4):325–32.
28. Li J, Brackbill RM, Stellman SD, Farfel MR, Miller-Archie SA, Friedman S, et al. Gastroesophageal reflux symptoms and comorbid asthma and posttraumatic stress disorder following the 9/11 terrorist attacks on world trade center in new York City. Am J Gastroenterol. 2011;106(11):1933–41.
29. Nair HP, Ekenga CC, Cone JE, Brackbill RM, Farfel MR, Stellman SD. Co-occurring lower respiratory symptoms and posttraumatic stress disorder 5 to 6 years after the world trade center terrorist attack. Am J Public Health. 2012;102(10):1964–73.
30. Stellman SD, Thomas PA, SO S, Brackbill RM, Farfel MR. Respiratory health of 985 children exposed to the world trade center disaster: report on world trade center health registry wave 2 follow-up, 2007-2008. J Asthma. 2013;50(4):354–63.
31. Szema AM, Savary KW, Ying BL, Lai K. Post 9/11: high asthma rates among children in Chinatown, New York. Allergy Asthma Proc. 2009;30(6):605–11.
32. Thomas PA, Brackbill R, Thalji L, DiGrande L, Campolucci S, Thorpe L, et al. Respiratory and other health effects reported in children exposed to the world trade center disaster of 11 September 2001. Environ Health Perspect. 2008;116(10):1383–90.
33. Reibman J, Liu M, Cheng Q, Liautaud S, Rogers L, Lau S, et al. Characteristics of a residential and working community with diverse exposure to world trade center dust, gas, and fumes. J Occup Environ Med. 2009;51(5):534–41.
34. Caplan-Shaw C, Kazeros A, Pradhan D, Berger K, Goldring R, Zhao S, et al. Improvement in severe lower respiratory symptoms and small airway function in world trade center dust exposed community members. Am J Ind Med. 2016;59(9):777–87.
35. Friedman SM, Farfel MR, Maslow CB, Cone JE, Brackbill RM, Stellman SD. Comorbid persistent lower respiratory symptoms and posttraumatic stress disorder 5–6 years post-9/11 in responders enrolled in the world trade center health registry. Am J Ind Med. 2013;56(11):1251–61.

36. Gross R, Neria Y, Tao XG, Massa J, Ashwell L, Davis K, et al. Posttraumatic stress disorder and other psychological sequelae among world trade center clean up and recovery workers. Ann N Y Acad Sci. 2006;1071:495–9.
37. Luft BJ, Schechter C, Kotov R, Broihier J, Reissman D, Guerrera K, et al. Exposure, probable PTSD and lower respiratory illness among world trade center rescue, recovery and clean-up workers. Psychol Med. 2012;42(5):1069–79.
38. Niles JK, Webber MP, Gustave J, Cohen HW, Zeig-Owens R, Kelly KJ, et al. Comorbid trends in world trade center cough syndrome and probable posttraumatic stress disorder in firefighters. Chest. 2011;140(5):1146–54.
39. Jordan HT, Stellman SD, Reibman J, Farfel MR, Brackbill RM, Friedman SM, et al. Factors associated with poor control of 9/11-related asthma 10-11 years after the 2001 world trade center terrorist attacks. J Asthma. 2015;52(6):630–7.
40. Friedman SM, Farfel MR, Maslow C, Jordan HT, Li J, Alper H, et al. Risk factors for and consequences of persistent lower respiratory symptoms among world trade center health registrants 10 years after the disaster. Occup Environ Med. 2016;73(10):676–84.
41. Hankinson JL, Odencrantz JR, Fedan KB. Spirometric reference values from a sample of the general U.S. population. Am J Respir Crit Care Med. 1999;159(1):179–87.
42. Crowley LE, Herbert R, Moline JM, Wallenstein S, Shukla G, Schechter C, et al. "Sarcoid like" granulomatous pulmonary disease in world trade center disaster responders. Am J Ind Med. 2011;54(3):175–84.
43. Izbicki G, Chavko R, Banauch GI, Weiden MD, Berger KI, Aldrich TK, et al. World trade center "sarcoid-like" granulomatous pulmonary disease in new York City fire Department rescue workers. Chest. 2007;131(5):1414–23.
44. Liu M, Qian M, Cheng Q, Berger KI, Shao Y, Turetz M, et al. Longitudinal spirometry among patients in a treatment program for community members with world trade center-related illness. J Occup Environ Med. 2012;54(10):1208–13.
45. Berger KI, Reibman J, Oppenheimer BW, Vlahos I, Harrison D, Goldring RM. Lessons from the world trade center disaster: airway disease presenting as restrictive dysfunction. Chest. 2013;144(1):249–57.
46. Kazeros A, Maa MT, Patrawalla P, Liu M, Shao Y, Qian M, et al. Elevated peripheral eosinophils are associated with new-onset and persistent wheeze and airflow obstruction in world trade center-exposed individuals. J Asthma. 2013;50(1):25–32.
47. Contoli M, Bousquet J, Fabbri LM, Magnussen H, Rabe KF, Siafakas NM, et al. The small airways and distal lung compartment in asthma and COPD: a time for reappraisal. Allergy. 2010;65(2):141–51.
48. Mead J. The lung's "quiet zone". N Engl J Med. 1970;282(23):1318–9.
49. Hewitt DJ. Interpretation of the "positive" methacholine challenge. Am J Ind Med. 2008;51(10):769–81.
50. Friedman SM, Maslow CB, Reibman J, Pillai PS, Goldring RM, Farfel MR, et al. Am J Respir Crit Care Med. 2011;184(5):582–9.
51. Oppenheimer BW, Goldring RM, Herberg ME, Hofer IS, Reyfman PA, Liautaud S, et al. Distal airway function in symptomatic subjects with normal spirometry following world trade center dust exposure. Chest. 2007;132(4):1275–82.
52. Berger KI, Turetz M, Liu M, Shao Y, Kazeros A, Parsia S, et al. Oscillometry complements spirometry in evaluation of subjects following toxic inhalation. ERJ Open Res. 2015;1(2):00043–2015.
53. Berger KI, Kalish S, Shao Y, Marmor M, Kazeros A, Oppenheimer BW, et al. Am J Ind Med. 2016;59(9):767–76.
54. Kazeros A, Zhang E, Cheng X, Shao Y, Liu M, Qian M, et al. Systemic inflammation associated with world trade center dust exposure and airways abnormalities in the local community. J Occup Environ Med. 2015;57(6):610–6.
55. Mendelson DS, Roggeveen M, Levin SM, Herbert R, de la Hoz RE. Air trapping detected on end-expiratory high-resolution computed tomography in symptomatic world trade center rescue and recovery workers. J Occup Environ Med. 2007;49(8):840–5.

56. Weiden MD, Ferrier N, Nolan A, Rom WN, Comfort A, Gustave J, et al. Obstructive airways disease with air trapping among firefighters exposed to world trade center dust. Chest. 2010;137(3):566–74.

57. Rom WN, Weiden M, Garcia R, Yie TA, Vathesatogkit P, Tse DB, et al. Acute eosinophilic pneumonia in a new York City firefighter exposed to world trade center dust. Am J Respir Crit Care Med. 2002;166(6):797–800.

58. Fireman EM, Lerman Y, Ganor E, Greif J, Fireman-Shoresh S, Lioy PJ, et al. Induced sputum assessment in new York City firefighters exposed to world trade center dust. Environ Health Perspect. 2004;112(15):1564–9.

59. Mann JM, Sha KK, Kline G, Breuer FU, Miller A. World trade center dyspnea: bronchiolitis obliterans with functional improvement: a case report. Am J Ind Med. 2005;48(3):225–9.

60. Wu M, Gordon RE, Herbert R, Padilla M, Moline J, Mendelson D, et al. Case report: lung disease in world trade center responders exposed to dust and smoke: carbon nanotubes found in the lungs of world trade center patients and dust samples. Environ Health Perspect. 2010;118(4):499–504.

61. Caplan-Shaw CE, Yee H, Rogers L, Abraham JL, Parsia SS, Naidich DP, et al. Lung pathologic findings in a local residential and working community exposed to world trade center dust, gas, and fumes. J Occup Environ Med. 2011;53(9):981–91.

62. Parsia SS, Yee H, Young S, et al. Characteristics of sarcoidosis in residents and workers exposed to world trade center dust, gas and fumes presenting for medical care. Am J Respir Crit Care Med. 2010;181:A1740.

Asthma in Children from New York City's Chinatown Post-9/11

Anthony M. Szema

Introduction

Asthma diagnoses in the pediatric population of Manhattan's Chinatown increased 50% in the year after September 11, 2001. Peak expiratory flow rates were reduced for those previously-diagnosed asthmatics living within 5 miles of Ground Zero, with increased asthma medication use and visits to the pediatrician for asthma. Years later, spirometry values for those alive in the neighborhood on 9/11, those born on 9/11, and those born thereafter are all reduced. The ongoing ambient air pollution with airborne metals suggests a two hit hypothesis with 9/11 plus post-9/11 air pollution,

A.M. Szema
Columbia University Child and Adolescent Psychiatric Epidemiology Group, CDC NIOSH U01 0H011308 "9/11 Trauma and Toxicity in Childhood: Longitudinal Health and Behavioral Outcomes", New York, NY, USA

Hofstra Northwell School of Medicine at Hofstra University, Hempstead, NY, USA

Department of Medicine, Division of Pulmonary and Critical Care, Northwell Health, Manhasset, NY, USA

Department of Medicine, Division of Allergy/Immunology, Northwell Health, Manhasset, NY, USA

Department of Occupational Medicine, Epidemiology, and Prevention, Northwell Health, Manhasset, NY, USA

Stony Brook University Department of Technology and Society, College of Engineering and Applied Sciences, Stony Brook, NY, USA

RDS2 Solutions, Stony Brook, NY, USA

Three Village Allergy & Asthma, PLLC, Stony Brook, NY, USA
e-mail: aszema@northwell.edu; anthony.szema@stonybrook.edu

© Springer International Publishing AG 2018
A.M. Szema (ed.), *World Trade Center Pulmonary Diseases and Multi-Organ System Manifestations*, DOI 10.1007/978-3-319-59372-2_5

the latter likely related to traffic over the Manhattan Bridge. These studies and those by Trasande suggest a need for long-term monitoring of this vulnerable population.

From the 2000 United States Census, serendipitously collected just 1 year prior to September 11, 2011, we were able to determine the rate of asthma in New York City's Chinese–American households was only 6.8%—among the lowest of all ten ethnic groups surveyed in NYC. Rosenbaum et al. reported that among these New York households in 2000 with at least one case of asthma, other Asian ethnicities had much higher rates of 11.7%: Korean, Japanese, Filipino, Vietnamese, and other Pacific Islanders. Other ethnicities ranged from a low of 7.3% (Asian Indian) to a high of 28% (Puerto Rican) (Fig. 1) [1]. Yet, the number of children with asthma in Chinatown increased 50% in the year post-9/11 [2].

The substantial increase in asthma among children in Chinatown after the World Trade Center disaster may be attributed to airborne hazards causing lung injury, which may clinically interpreted as asthma. Air pollution may irritate and inflame airways, leading to cardinal features of asthma: airway hyperresponsiveness and inflammation. Samples of signature World Trade Center dust, collected after falling to the ground in the vicinity by Paul Lioy on September 16 and 17, 2001, included calcium, phthalate esters, plastic, combusted jet fuel, soot, inorganic metals, radionuclides, ionic species, and asbestos (0.8% to 3% of the mass) [3]. All of these particulates are known hazards to the lung.

The satellite photo from the International Space Station shows Chinatown directly affected by the plume which headed east (Fig. 2). Manhattan's Chinatown, seen in a local map, is blocks from the Twin Towers site (Fig. 3).

NYC Households With At Least One Person With Asthma (2000 Census data)

• Non-Hispanic white	11.0
• Non-Hispanic black	15.8
• Puerto Rican	28.0
• Dominican	14.8
• Central/South American	13.0
• Mexican	5.0
• Other Hispanic (Cuban)	16.8
• Chinese	6.8
• Asian Indian	7.3
• Other Asian	11.7

Other Asian comprises Korean, Japanese, Filipino, Vietnamese, and other pacific Islanders)

Fig. 1 NYC households with at least one person with asthma (2000 US Census Data) from [1]

Fig. 2 Satellite photo of New York City on September 11, 2001, which shows plume of smoke from the burning World Trade Center enveloping Chinatown, Manhattan (from International Space Station downloaded from globalsecurity.org with permission)

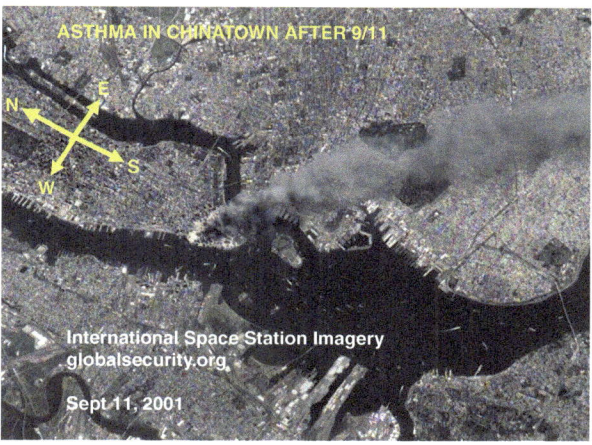

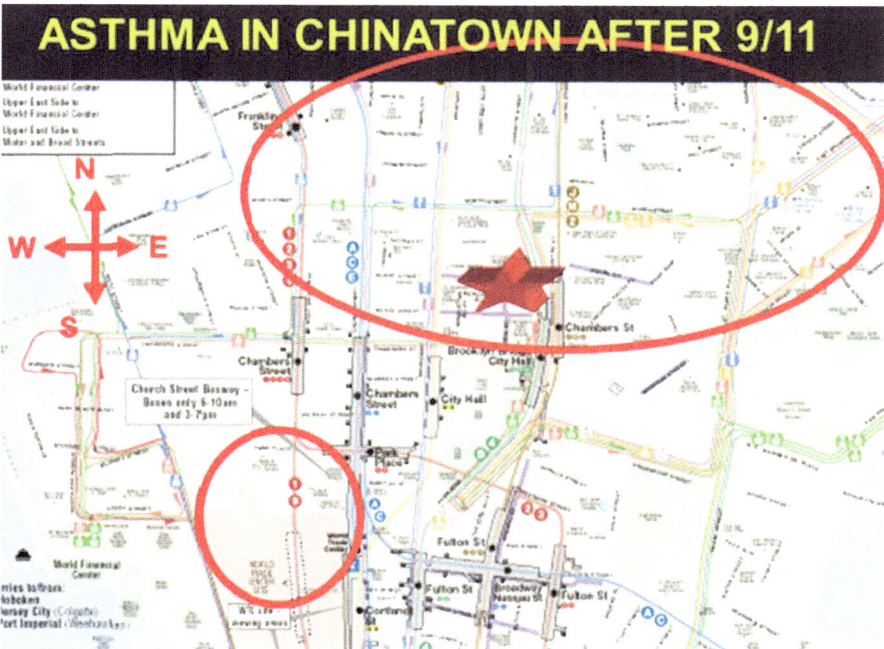

Fig. 3 New York City map shows proximity of the Chinatown Manhattan neighborhood to the World Trade Center Twin Towers, and the closest border is three blocks away

What our team found specifically was that Chinese–American children enrolled in an Asthma Registry and living in Chinatown, blocks away from Ground Zero, had more asthma-related clinic visits post-9/11 compared to the prior twelve months. Asthmatic children living within 5 miles of the World Trade Center site had more clinic visits than those living more than 5 miles away (Fig. 4). There were more prescriptions for asthma medications.

Whereas in the 12 months following the 9/11 attacks, new cases of asthma increased 50% in Manhattan's Chinatown, cases decreased 11.9% in Queen's Chinatown (aka Flushing) approximately 12 miles away. Both groups comprised urban, lower socioeconomic strata Chinese–American children treated by the same salaried physicians.

Mean percent predicted peak expiratory flow rates decreased solely for those patients living within 5 miles of Ground Zero after September 11, 2001 (Fig. 5). All values in Region 2 shown in yellow (which is greater than 5 miles from Ground

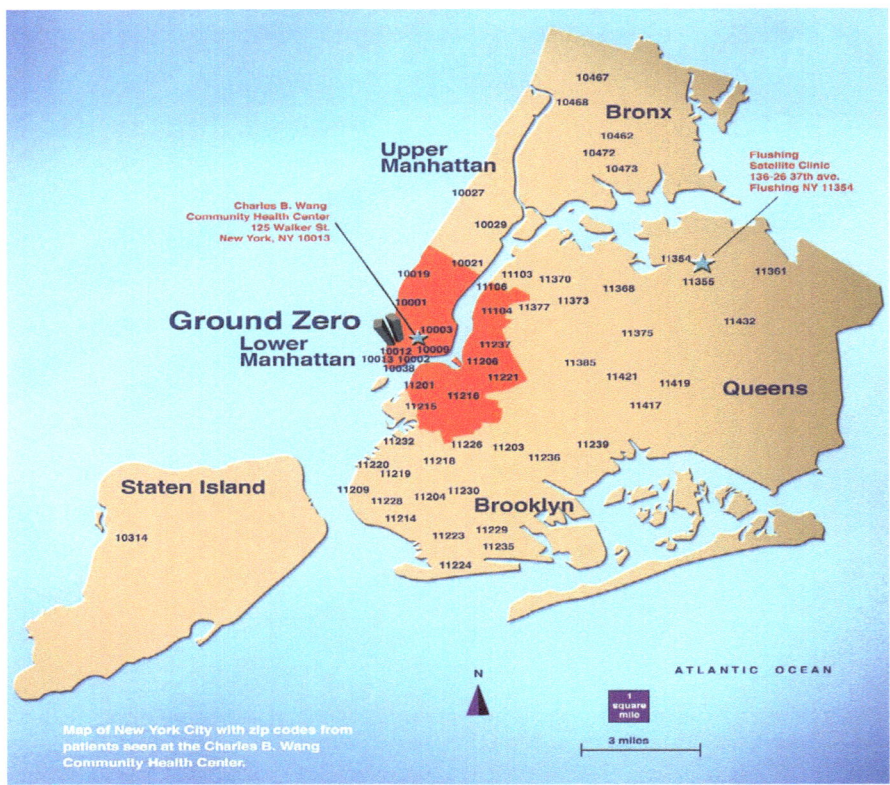

Fig. 4 Map of NYC shows zip codes of children living within 5 miles of Ground Zero in *red* compared to those living beyond 5 miles. *Blue stars* indicate locations of the clinics where children were examined. Zip codes in *red* are in zone 1 (<5 miles from the Twin Towers of the World Trade Center), while zip codes in tan are for those New York City zip codes greater than 5 miles away [2]

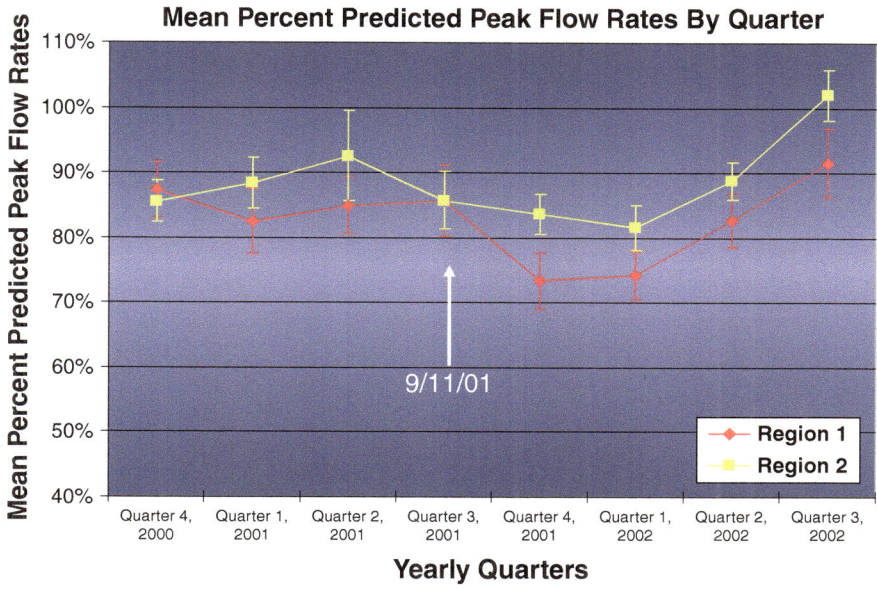

Fig. 5 Reduction in Peak Flow Rates for those students living within 5 miles of WTC [2]

Zero) were within normal limits (greater than 80% predicted) throughout the 2-year study period. In Region 1 shown in red, however, values fell below normal (73.4%) for the quarter following 9/11/01 and gradually returned to baseline (within the normal range) two quarters after the disaster.

Lin et al. found self-reported asthma rates among 476 second graders at four Chinatown elementary school students to be 16% in 2005 and 21.6% in 2006. Redline screening questionnaire data yielded rates of 46.1% and 52%, respectively [4]. So, these data support the concept that asthma rates are now persistently high in Chinatown children post-9/11.

Our study population comprised 1000 students attending the closest, ethnically and socioeconomically homogeneous elementary school proximal to the World Trade Center. Deployed on the roof of the school, 14 m above ground, were two fine particulate sampler monitors installed by the New York State Department of Environmental Conservation. These monitors sampled 2.5 μm-sized particulate mass samples collected continuously every 3 days (Fig. 6). We distributed a questionnaire to parents and students (Redline asthma questionnaire) [5] (Figs. 7, 8, 9, and 10) and also obtained demographic information, age, gender, height, weight, presence of household smokers, use of asthma medications, diagnosis of asthma by a pediatrician, and alternative medicine (herbal, moxibustion) for asthma. Spirometry required parental consent and student assent; we used the KoKo Legend Spirometer. Spirometry calibrated daily and results adjusted for temperature, barometric pressure, age, height, gender, and race. A minimum of eight forced vital capacity (FVC) maneuvers were performed to achieve three acceptable flow-volume loops

Fig. 6 Particulate sampler
monitor installed by the
New York State Department
of Environmental
Conservation

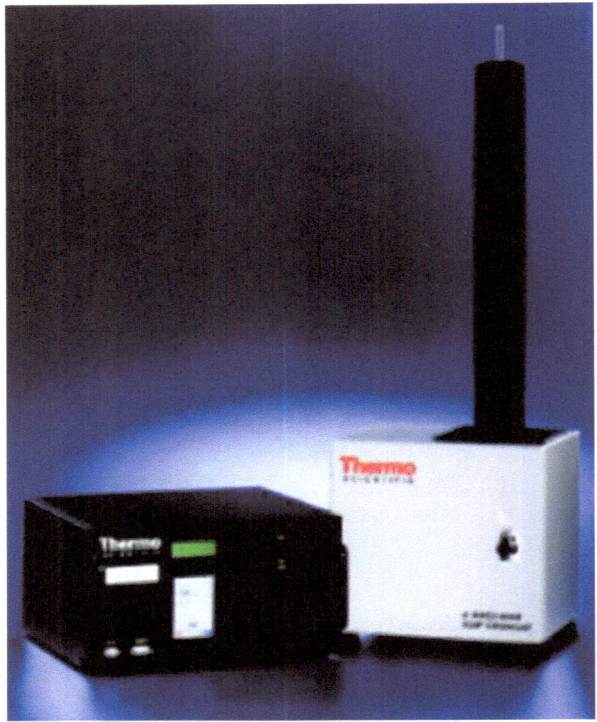

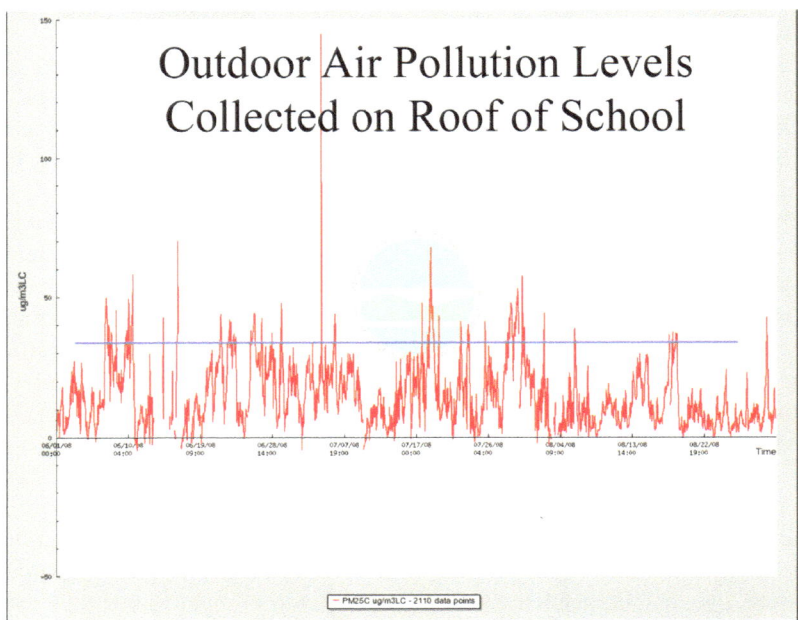

Fig. 7 Outdoor air pollution levels collected on the roof of the school. Outdoor air pollution levels
frequently exceeded Environmental Protection Agency (EPA) limits 35 μg/m³/24 h (*blue line*) [9].
Data supplied by David Wheeler, New York State Department of Environmental Conservation

STUDENT QUESTIONNAIRE

Name _____ Age _____ Grade _____ Teacher _____

Race ☐ African American ☐ Asian American ☐ Hispanic ☐ White ☐ Native American ☐ Other

Please tell us how often you have any of the following:

		NEVER	SOMETIMES	A LOT
1.	My breathing sounds noisy or wheezy	o	o	O
2.	It is hard to take a deep breath	o	o	O
3.	It is hard for me to stop coughing	o	o	O
4.	My chest feels tight or hurts after I run, play hard, or do sports.	o	o	O
5.	I wake up at night coughing	o	o	O
6.	I wake up at night because I have trouble breathing	o	o	O
7.	I cough when I run, climb stairs or play sports.	o	o	O
8.	My eyes get itchy, puffy or burn	o	o	O
9.	I have problems with a runny or stuffy nose	o	o	O

Please answer the following questions

		YES	NO
10.	A doctor or nurse told me that I have asthma.	O	O
11.	I stayed in the hospital overnight for asthma or trouble breathing this past year.	O	O
12.	I take medicine or use an inhaler for asthma.	O	O
13.	I take medicine for allergies.	O	O

Fig. 8 Redline questionnaire for asthma

with two being within 200 mL for FVC and forced expiratory volume at 1 s (FEV1). The value assigned to a participant was the largest acceptable value within 200 mL of a second value [6–8].

We received 353 questionnaires from parents of children at an elementary school in Chinatown.

We conducted spirometry on 202 students.

Using a DUSTREAM™ vacuum collection system, dust from around the school was collected and sent to Indoor Biotechnologies (Charlottesville, VA) [10] for analysis by ELISA for concentrations of antigens:

PARENT OR GUARDIAN QUESTIONNAIRE

Student's Name _____ Age ____ Grade ____ Teacher _____
Student's Race ☐ African American ☐ Asian American ☐ Hispanic ☐ White ☐ Native American ☐ Other

Please tell us how often your child has any of the following. (If your child has more problems in some seasons of the year, please tell us about problems during the worst season.) Does your child ...

		NEVER	SOMETIMES	A LOT	Don't Know
1	Make noisy or wheezy sounds when breathing?	O	O	O	☐
2	Have a hard time taking a deep breath?	O	O	O	☐
3	Develop coughs that won't go away?	O	O	O	☐
4	Complain about a chest that feels tight or hurts after running, playing hard, or doing sports?	O	O	O	☐
5	Wake up at night coughing?	O	O	O	☐
6	Wake up at night because of trouble breathing?	O	O	O	☐
7	Cough when running, climbing stairs or playing sports?	O	O	O	☐
8	Miss days of school (absent from school) because of breathing problems?	O	O	O	☐
9	Have eyes that itch, get puffy or burn	O	O	O	☐
10	Have problems with a runny, stuffy nose	O	O	O	☐

Please answer the following questions about your child:

		YES	NO	Don't Know
11	Has a doctor or nurse told you that your child has asthma, reactive airway disease or wheezy bronchitis?	O	O	☐
12	Has your child stayed in the hospital overnight for asthma or for trouble breathing this past year?	O	O	☐
13	Does your child take medicine (or use an inhaler) for asthma?	O	O	☐
14	Does your child take medicine for allergies?	O	O	☐

Fig. 9 Parental questionnaire regarding their child's asthma

– Mouse
– Rat
– Feline (cat)
– Cockroach
– Three groups of dust mites
– Dog

Undetectable of extremely low levels of these indoor aeroallergens supports a lack of a role for specific allergic sensitization to these common indoor triggers of asthma (Fig. 11).

家長或監護人問卷調查（7歲以下小孩）

學生姓名 ____________ 年齡 _____ 年級 _____ 教師姓名 ____________

學生種族: 非洲美國人 亞洲美國人 西班牙裔美國人 白人 其他

請告訴我們你有否注意到你孩子有以下情況。(如果你的孩子在學期本節沒有發生特別的問題，請告訴我們在學期的本節沒有發生問題。) 你的孩子有.....

	從來沒有	有時	最多	不知道
1. 呼吸不暢順或有雜音嗎?	○	○	○	□
2. 深呼吸困難嗎?	○	○	○	□
3. 是否有長時間性的咳嗽?	○	○	○	□
4. 在跑完步玩得興奮或運動完之後，感到胸口緊或不舒服嗎?	○	○	○	□
5. 在半夜因咳嗽而醒來嗎?	○	○	○	□
6. 因呼吸不順而導致半夜起床嗎?	○	○	○	□
7. 在跑步，爬樓梯或運動時咳嗽嗎?	○	○	○	□
8. 因呼吸道的問題而不上學（缺席）嗎?	○	○	○	□
9. 覺得眼睛痕癢，紅腫，刺痛嗎?	○	○	○	□
10. 流鼻涕或鼻塞的問題嗎?	○	○	○	□

請回答以下有關於你孩子的問題:

11. 是否曾經有醫生或護士有告訴過你，你孩子有哮喘病?	○ 是	○ 否	□ 不知道
12. 在過去的一年，你孩子是否曾經因哮喘病或呼吸性疾病而住院?	○ 是	○ 否	□ 不知道
13. 你孩子是否服用哮喘病藥物或使用哮喘噴霧器?	○ 是	○ 否	□ 不知道
14. 你孩子有否因過敏而服用藥物嗎?	○ 有	○ 否	□ 不知道

Fig. 10 Parental asthma questionnaire translated into Chinese

Among children who answered questionnaires but refused spirometry, 12.6% of those living within 1 mile of Ground Zero self-reported asthma vs. 4.8% for those living further away (Fig. 12).

Mite Allergens			Cat	Dog	Cockroach	Rat	Mouse
Der p 1	Per f 1	Mite Group 2	Fel d 1	Can f 1	Bla g 2	Rat n 1	Mus m 1
0	0	0	0.31	0	0	0	0.068

Fig. 11 Undetectable and insignificant levels of indoor aeroallergens in dust from an elementary school in Chinatown [6]

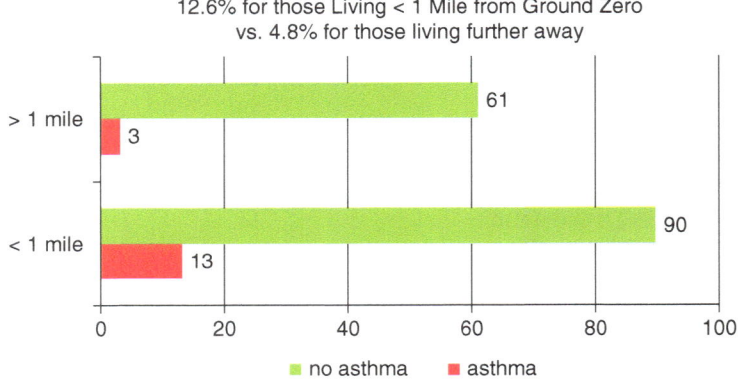

Self-Reported Asthma Rates Among Students Without Spirometry

12.6% for those Living < 1 Mile from Ground Zero vs. 4.8% for those living further away

■ no asthma ■ asthma

Fig. 12 Higher self-reported asthma rates among children living within 1 mile of Ground Zero who refused spirometry

Fig. 13 Rates of asthma higher for children living > 1 mile away

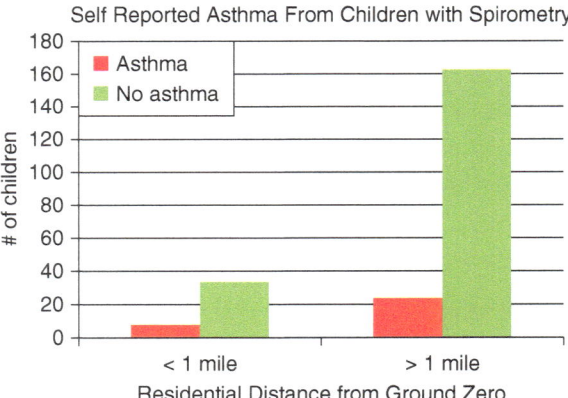

Self Reported Asthma From Children with Spirometry

■ Asthma
■ No asthma

# of children

Residential Distance from Ground Zero

For those children who underwent spirometry, rates of asthma were actually higher for those living more than 1 mile away. However, there are more children living further away (Fig. 13).

Post 9/11: High asthma rates among children in Chinatown, NY

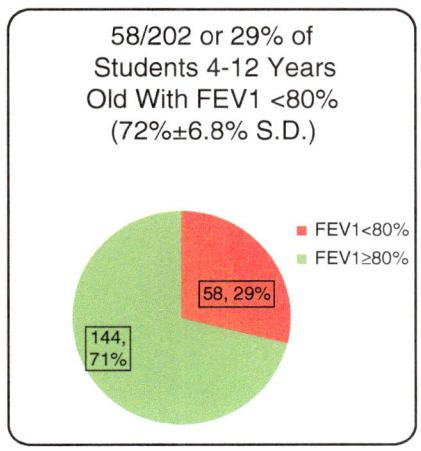

58/202 or 29% of Students 4-12 Years Old With FEV1 <80% (72%±6.8% S.D.)

■ FEV1<80%
■ FEV1≥80%

58, 29%

144, 71%

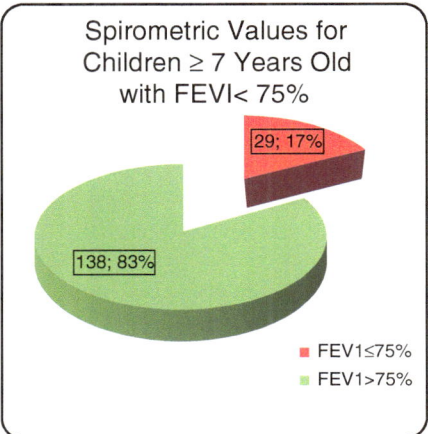

Spirometric Values for Children ≥ 7 Years Old with FEVl< 75%

29; 17%

138; 83%

■ FEV1≤75%
■ FEV1>75%

Fig. 14 Children born on 9/11 had a 17% airway obstruction rate, while 29% of those alive on 9/11 exhibited airway obstruction

Fig. 15 Impulse Oscillometry (IOS) from Jaeger Carefusion Website

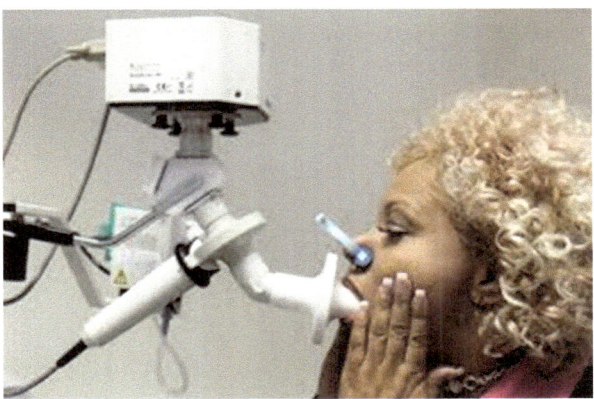

For those children alive on 9/11 (≥7 years old in 2008), 17% had airway obstruction with FEV1 < 75%. For those students born after 9/11, 29% had an FEV1 < 80% (Fig. 14) [6].

Chinatown asthma rates are therefore still higher than other groups (29% vs. the NYC reference rate of 13%). These rates indicate persistence of elevated rates, as suggested by Lin and colleagues. Air pollution levels exceed EPA standards and are unhealthy (>25 µg/m³/day). This ongoing air pollution may account for increased asthma incidence in children living in Manhattan's Chinatown whether they were alive on 9/11 or born thereafter. It is possible that exposure to various toxins on 9/11 accentuated the effect of subsequent exposure to air pollution.

The difference between parent-reported prevalence of asthma (12.6%) and tested prevalence (29% overall) corresponds to those reported by the Harlem Children's Zone Asthma Initiative and suggests a high degree of unmet need for asthma treatment and lower-than-necessary child well-being and health status [6].

We next measured impulse oscillometry (IOS) of the small airways as a measure of peripheral airways lung function and airway hyperresponsiveness. IOS can be used to determine geographic location of airways narrowing, distal vs. proximal, as well as airway hyperresponsiveness. One hundred and fifty-eight students completed Redline questionnaires (Fig. 8) with their parents (Fig. 9) and 129 completed impulse oscillometry (Fig. 15). We also analyzed speciated air pollution data for metal content.

A Jaeger MasterScreen impulse oscillometry system (CareFusion Germany 234 GmbH) was loaned by CareFusion Corporation, and training was provided by Steven Spungen, M.S. The IOS requires three trials of 20 s each to take 100 complete measurements. A loudspeaker delivers pulse-shaped pressure flow excitation to the respiratory system. The overall impedance of the pulse is due to the resistive and viscoelastic forces of the respiratory system. IOS is reported as resistance and reactance measured in cm of water per liter per second. The Jaeger IOS was calibrated with a reference resistor (2 cm $H_2O/L/s$) according to the manufacturer's instructions. Multifrequency impulses were applied over 20 s trials to the airway through the mouthpiece during tidal breathing. Children used a noseclip. Three reproducible trials were obtained if they lacked artifacts from coughing, breath holding, swallowing, or vocalization.

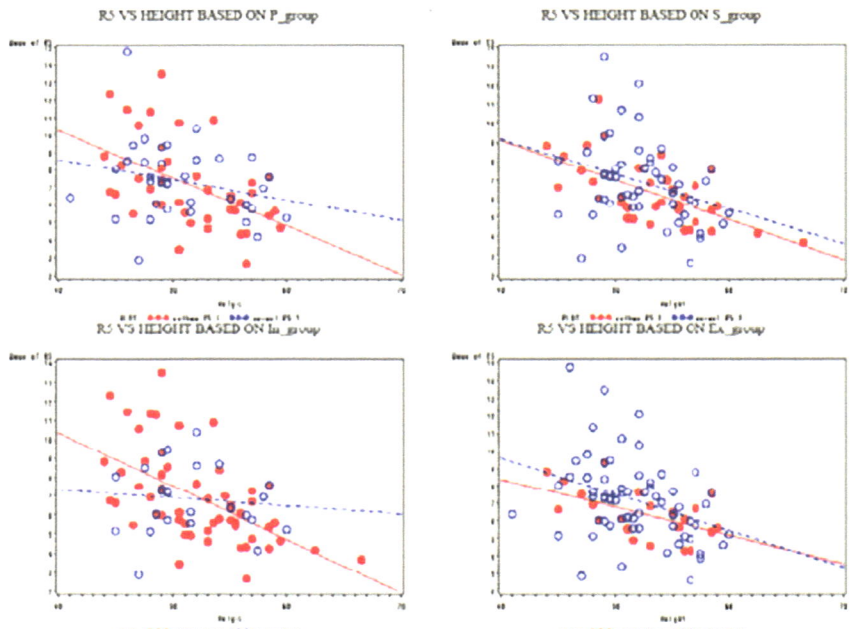

Fig. 16 R5 values appropriate for height and linearly correlated

Allergy and respiratory symptoms are common among those children (confirmed by parents) responding to the survey distributed among classrooms at the closest elementary school to the World Trade Center site. There were strong correlations between responses from children and their parents (Fig. 16). Frequent severe symptoms such as wheezing and chest tightness, juxtaposed with use of allergy and asthma medications, support the concept that these patients are not clinically well controlled. Boys and girls in this cohort had increased values of airway resistance at 5 Hz, with boys having higher values than girls (Figs. 17 and 18). Frequency

Correlations of Parent and Child Responses for Asthma and All Allergy Symptoms from the Validation Sample*(n = 158)

Student Question# (Paired with Parent Questions**)	Sample Size	Responses Spearman r	Two-sided P value
Making noisy sounds or wheezing (1)	87	0.748	<0.001
Hard to take a deep breath (2)	84	0.895	<0.001
Hard to stop coughing (3)	90	0. 646	<0.001
Chest feels tight after run (4)	85	0.880	<0.001
Wake up at night coughing (5)	93	0.749	<0.001
Wake up at night because of Trouble breathing (6)	87	0.713	<0.001
Cough when climbing stairs (7)	85	0.738	<0.001
Have eyes itch, get puffy (8)	89	0.870	<0.001
Have problems with a runny, Stuffy nose (9)	89	0.824	<0.001
A doctor or nurse told me that I have asthma (10)	89	0.935	<0.001
Stayed in hospital overnight (11) * **			
Take medicine for asthma (12)	90	0.848	<0.001
Take medicine for allergies (13)	93	0.832	<0.001

Fig. 17 Strong correlation between parental and child surveys for asthma symptoms

Table1 (n = 114)

Variables	Boys(57) Means ± SD	Girls(57) Means ± SD
Age(year)	8.20±1.86	8.35±1.79
Height(cm)	131.57±11.65	132.28±11.08
Weight(kg)	31.24±8.92	30.08±8.66
Mean_R5	7.24±2.14	6.74±2.28
Mean_R20	3.42±1.13	3.28±0.80
Mean_x5	−2.77±2.58	−2.74±2.94

When comparing boys higher vs. girls

Fig. 18 R5-R20 is a measure of distal airways narrowing and is higher in boys vs. girls. Mean R5, X5, and R20 (resistance at 5 Hz, reactance at 5 Hz, and resistance at 20 Hz, respectively) given in centimeters of H20 per liter per second were high. Boys and girls with average ages of 8 years, height of 132 cm, and weight 31 kg, had: boys values of R5 = 7.2, X5 = −2, and R20 = 3; and girls values of R5 = 6.7, X5 = −2.7, and R20 = 3.2. Mean values for the entire group of boys and girls were R5 = 6.99, X5 = −2.75, and R20 = 3.35. *R5* resistance at 5 Hz, *X5* reactance at 5 Hz, *R20* resistance at 20 Hz. ±IOS measurements are given in centimeters of H_2O per liter per second, except for resonant frequency, which is given in Hertz. IOS measurements are given as resistance and reactance at 5 and 20 Hz

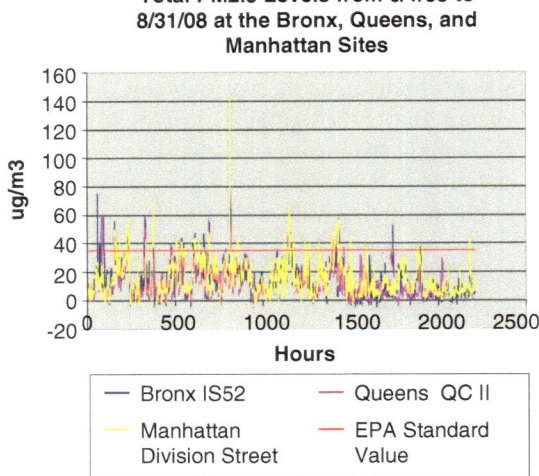

Fig. 19 Air pollution levels at several NYC sites compared to school (Manhattan Division Street)

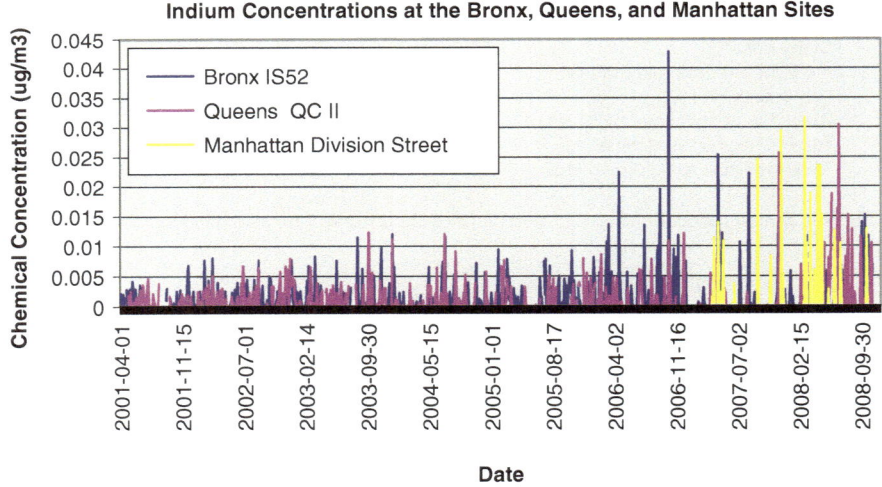

Fig. 20 Indium concentrations in air

dependence between resistance values at 5 Hz and 20 Hz suggest small airways dysfunction rather than central airways narrowing. Air pollution levels are high and contain detectable lead, vanadium, and indium (Figs. 19, 20, 21, and 22).

Trasande et al. performed a cross-sectional study of 148 children who were <18 years old on September 11, 2001, and presented to the World Trade Center Environmental Health Center/Survivors Health Program. In this cohort, 38.5% were caught in the dust cloud from the collapsing buildings on September 11; over 80% spent ≥1 day in their home between September 11 and 18, 2001, and 25.7% reported home dust exposure. New-onset nasal/sinus congestion was reported in 52.7%, while nearly one-third reported new gastroesophageal reflux (GERD) symptoms.

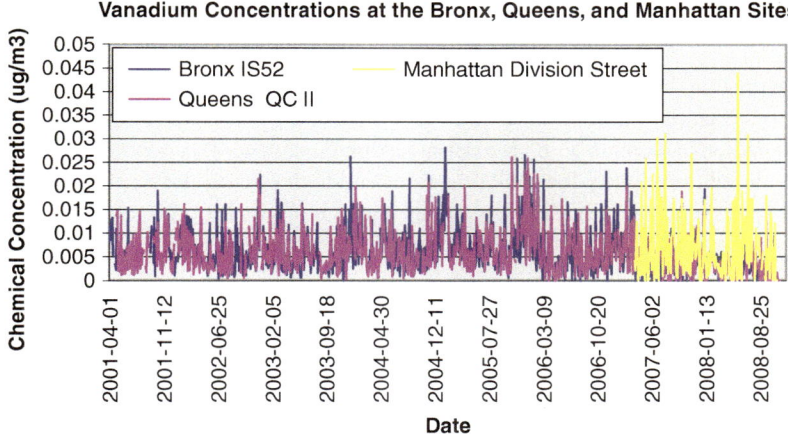

Fig. 21 Vanadium air concentrations

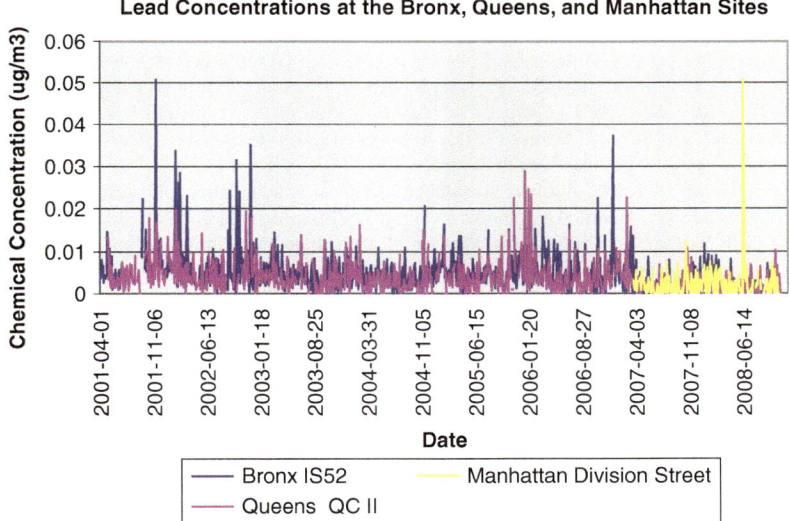

Fig. 22 Lead air concentrations

Multivariable regression with exposure variables, body mass index category, and age as covariates identified strongest associations of dust cloud with spirometry (17.1% decrease in maximum midexpiratory flow). Younger children experienced increased peripheral eosinophils (+0.098% per year, $p = 0.023$), while older children experienced more new-onset GERD (OR 1.17, $p = 0.004$), headaches (OR 1.10, $p = 0.011$), and prehypertension (OR 1.09, $p = 0.024$). Home dust exposure was associated with reduced high-density lipoprotein (-10.3 mg/dL, $p = 0.027$) and elevated triglycerides (+36.3 mg/dL, $p = 0.033$). These data concur not only with our findings but also suggest the need for more extensive study of respiratory, metabolic, and cardiovascular consequences [11].

Conclusion

In conclusion, the events of September 11, 2001, at the World Trade Center led to airborne hazards, increasing asthma rates in NYC's Chinatown and exacerbating those pediatric patients with preexisting asthma in a dose-dependent manner related to residential proximity for peak flow rates and high rates in the neighborhood overall. The persistence of high asthma rates and symptoms for those alive on 9/11 and the very high rates for those children born even after 9/11 suggests ongoing unmet pulmonary health care needs similar to that of the Harlem Children's Zone Asthma Initiative and 9/11 rescue workers [12–15].

References

1. Rosenbaum E. Racial/ethnic differences in asthma prevalence: the role of housing and neighborhood environments. J Health Soc Behav. 2008;49:131–45.
2. Szema AM, Khedkar M, Maloney PF, et al. Clinical deterioration in pediatric asthmatic patients after September 11, 2001. J Allergy Clin Immunol. 2004;113(3):420–6.
3. Lioy PJ, Weisel CP, Millette JR, Eisenreich S, Vallero D, Offenberg J, Buckley B, Turpin B, Zhong M, Cohen MD, Prophete C, Yang I, Stiles R, Chee G, Johnson W, Porcja R, Alimokhtari S, Hale RC, Weschler C, Chen LC. Characterization of the dust/smoke aerosol that settled east of the World Trade Center (WTC) in lower Manhattan after the collapse of the WTC 11 September 2001. Environ Health Perspect. 2002;110(7):703–14.
4. Lin DH, Au L, Ko D. Asthma prevalence in Lower Manhattan public primary schools. In: American Public Health Association meeting, Washington, DC, 3–7 Nov 2007.
5. Redline S, Gruchella RS, Wolf ML, et al. Development and validation of school-based asthma and allergy screening questionnaires in a 4-city study. Ann Allergy Asthma Immunol. 2004;93:36–48.
6. Szema A, Savary K, Ying B, Lai K. Post 9/11: high asthma rates in Manhattan's Chinatown, New York, AAP. 2009.
7. Brusasco V, Crapo R, Viegi G, editors. ATS/ERS task force: standardisation of lung function testing. Eur Respir J. 2005;26:319–538.
8. Polgar C, Promodhat V. Pulmonary function in children: techniques and standards. 3rd ed. Philadelphia, PA: WB Saunders; 1971.
9. Environmental Protection Agency. Final designations for the 24-hour Fine Particle Standard established in 2006. Available online at www.epa.gov./pmdesignations/2006standards/documents/2008-12-22/factsheet.htm. last Accessed 1 Sept 2009.
10. Earle CD, King EM, Tsay A, et al. High-throughput fluorescent multiplex array for indoor allergen exposure assessment. J Allergy Clin Immunol. 2007;119:428–33.
11. Trasande L, Fiorino EK, Attina T, Berger K, Goldring R, Chemtob C, Levy-Carrick N, Shao Y, Liu M, Urbina E, Reibman J. Associations of World Trade Center exposures with pulmonary and cardiometabolic outcomes among children seeking care for health concerns. Sci Total Environ. 2013;444:320–6.
12. Claudio L, Stingone JA, Godbold J. Prevalence of childhood asthma in urban communities: the impact of ethnicity and income. Ann Epidemiol. 2006;16:332–40.
13. Nicholas SW, Jean-Louis B, Ortiz B, et al. Addressing the childhood asthma crisis in Harlem: the Harlem children's zone asthma initiative. Am J Public Health. 2005;95:245–9.

14. Banauch GI, Izbicki G, Christodovlou V, et al. Pulmonary function after exposure to the world trade center collapse in the New York City Fire Department. Am J Respir Crit Care Med. 2006;174:312–9.

15. Banauch GI, Izbicki G, Christodovlou V, et al. Trial of prophylactic inhaled steroids to prevent or reduce pulmonary function decline, pulmonary symptoms, and airway hyperreactivity in firefighters at the world trade center site. Disaster Med Public Health Prep. 2008;2:33–9.

Cancer Risk Post 9/11

Elizabeth Ward

Introduction

Individuals caught in the dust cloud on 9/11 and working on or near the site in the days immediately following the attack experienced intense acute exposures to a mixture of substances whose concentration and composition will never be fully known. The dust was highly alkaline, due to pulverized cement, and contained numerous particles, fibers, and glass shards, soon resulting in eye, nose, and throat irritation and what came to be known as WTC cough [1]. Smoke from persistent fires contained polycyclic aromatic hydrocarbons, metals, and many other chemicals. Although levels of airborne contaminants were not measured in the first 4 days, the high prevalence of acute and chronic respiratory conditions in firefighters and rescue and cleanup workers amply documents significant exposure levels and toxicity [1]. Although some of the dust and smoke was carried away into higher levels of the atmosphere, significant amounts of dusts and smoke settled in surrounding streets, residences, and office buildings, creating substantial potential for chronic airborne exposure to resuspended dusts and dermal exposure through contact with contaminated surfaces.

Both responder populations and area residents and workers had potential for significant exposures to known and possible carcinogens present in the materials released from the WTC site (Table 1). The presence of these carcinogens raised the possibility that exposures related to the WTC collapse and fires could lead to an increased risk of cancer. The potential association between WTC exposures and cancer has been investigated in four WTC-exposed populations to date: firefighters employed by the Fire Department of New York (FDNY) [1], rescue and recovery

E. Ward
Intramural Research, American Cancer Society, 250 Williams St., Atlanta, GA 30303, USA
e-mail: eward04@gmail.com

© Springer International Publishing AG 2018
A.M. Szema (ed.), *World Trade Center Pulmonary Diseases and Multi-Organ System Manifestations*, DOI 10.1007/978-3-319-59372-2_6

Table 1 Carcinogens present in WTC dust and fume

Asbestos	Asbestos is designated as a known human carcinogen by IARC, with sufficient evidence for cancer of the larynx, lung, mesothelioma, and ovary and limited evidence for cancer of the colorectum, pharynx, and stomach. Bulk samples of outdoor dusts collected on September 16, 2001, on Cortland Street, Cherry Avenue, and Market Street, outside the perimeter of the WTC site, had 0.8–3% asbestos by weight [23]. The main source of asbestos was the chrysotile used to insulate the lower half of the first tower
Polycyclic aromatic hydrocarbons	Carcinogenic polycyclic aromatic hydrocarbons (PAHs) are produced by combustion of wood, coal, and any other carbonaceous material and are important causes of occupational lung cancer. The carcinogenicity of specific PAHs has been evaluated by IARC. Benzo(a)pyrene is listed by IARC in Group 1 (carcinogenic), dibenz[a,h]anthracene is listed in Group 2A (probably carcinogenic), and benz[a]anthracene, benzo[b] fluoranthene, and benzo[k]fluoranthene are listed in 2B (possibly carcinogenic). Sources of PAHs at the WTC included the burning of about 90,000 liters of jet fuel, 500,000 liters of transformer oil, 380,000 liters of fuel oil, and approximately the same amount of gasoline plus any and all burning items. Heavy machinery and power tool brought to the site added to particulate and PAH exposures
Polychlorinated biphenyls, chlorinated dioxins, furans	Polychlorinated biphenyls (PCBs) were present in the transformer oil in the electrical power substation s located in the World Trade Center, and dioxin-like compounds are formed when chlorinated plastics like PVC are burned. Polychlorinated biphenyls, dioxin-like, with a toxic equivalency factor (TEF) according to WHO (PCBs 77, 81, 105, 114, 118, 123, 126, 156, 157, 167, 169, 189), 2,3,7,8-tetrachlorodibenzo-para-dioxin, 2,3,4,7,8-pentachlorodibenzofuran, and 3,3′,4,4′,5-pentachlorobiphenyl, are classified by IARC as carcinogenic to humans (Group 1)
Particulates	A wide variety of particulates were generated from the building materials when the WTC collapsed, including silica, an IARC Group 1 carcinogen. Exposure to small particulates (PM less than 2.5 microns) in outdoor air pollution and air pollution from burning biomass in poorly ventilated cooking stoves has also been designated by IARC as known human carcinogens based on increased lung cancer in exposed population. Diesel exhaust was also generated by construction and transportation vehicles used at the site and is also designated as a known human carcinogen based on excess lung cancer in exposed occupational groups
Carcinogenic metals	Five metals (arsenic, beryllium, cadmium, chromium, and nickel) measured in WTC dust and air samples are listed as Group 1 carcinogens by IARC; all increase risk for lung cancer with other cancer sites of sufficient or limited evidence in humans varying by metal
Volatile organic compounds (VOCs)	Benzene, 1,3 butadiene, and formaldehyde are common exposures present in combustion products that are listed as Group 1 carcinogens by IARC

workers enrolled in the World Trade Center Health Program (WTCHP) health monitoring program [2, 3], WTC registry enrollees (rescue and recovery workers and community survivors) [4, 5], and police officers employed by the New York City Police Department [7]. A systematic review of the methods and results of three of the studies on cancer incidence in rescue and recovery workers has also been published [8].

Fire Department of New York (FDNY) Firefighters

A cancer incidence study was conducted among 9853 men who were employed as firefighters on Jan 1, 1996, 8927 of whom had exposure to the WTC site [2]. The cancer experience of all firefighters before 9/11 and nonexposed firefighters after 9/11 was used as an internal control population. Cancers diagnosed before the study end date (12/31/2008) were identified through linkage with state cancer registries in New York and four other states where the majority of retirees live and self-reported cases were confirmed from medical records. The expected number of cancer cases, adjusted for age, race, and ethnic origin, and secular trends was calculated separately for exposed and nonexposed person-years using SEER Registry rates as the referent. The standardized incidence ratios (SIRs) for exposed person time and the ratios of SIRs for nonexposed and exposed person time were the primary outcome measures. Additional analyses included corrections for potential surveillance bias and modified cohort inclusion criteria.

The study found that the standard incidence ratio (SIR) for cancers of all sites in exposed firefighters was 1.10 (95% CI, 0.98–1.25) and the SIR for exposed vs. nonexposed person time was 1.32 (95% CI, 1.07–1.62). There were no significant excesses for specific cancers; however, the SIR for exposed compared to unexposed person-years was greater than 1.00 for 10 of 15 cancers examined. Given the relatively small numbers of total cancers identified among exposed firefighters, the expected number of cancers for most specific sites was small, and the study had limited statistical power to detect excesses. The study found no evidence of an exposure-response gradient on the basis of either FDNY arrival time or the common WTC exposure categories.

World Trade Center Health Program (WTCHP) Enrollees

A cancer incidence study was conducted among WTC responders enrolled in the World Trade Center Health Program (WTCHP) [2]. The WTCHP provides medical monitoring and treatment for individuals who participated (as employees and/or volunteers) in the rescue, recovery, and cleanup efforts at Ground Zero (WTC responders). Medical monitoring and treatment for responders is one of the four programs administered by NIOSH to provide services to 9/11-affected populations; the others include FDNY firefighters, survivors of Pentagon, and Shanksville, PA, responders. Eligibility for enrollment in the WTC responder program, which remains open, is based on the type of duties, site location, and dates and hours worked. In addition to medical monitoring, treatment is provided for responders who develop WTC-related conditions.

A cancer incidence study was conducted in 20,984 responders enrolled in the WTCHP from July 16, 2002 to December 31, 2008 [2]. Cancer case identification was performed through linkage with the state tumor registries of New York, New Jersey, Connecticut, and Pennsylvania, which account for 98% of the residences for responders at time of enrollment. Self-reported exposures were categorized based on four variables: occupation, extent of exposure to the dust cloud on 9/11, duration working at the site, and work on the debris pile during four time periods (September 2001, October 2001, November–December 2001, January–June 2002) [6]. An integrated exposure variable was created using a 4-point scale (very high, high, intermediate, and low) based on total time spent working at Ground Zero, exposure to the dust cloud, and work on the debris pile [10]. Vital status was obtained through linkage with the National Death Index and next-of-kin reports. Person-years at risk were censored at the time of death or December 31, 2008, whichever came sooner. Expected numbers of cancer cases were calculated based on state rates (New York, New Jersey, and Connecticut) and national rates (Pennsylvania). The SIR among registrant "responders" was elevated and statistically significant for all cancer sites combined (SIR = 1.15; 95% CI, 1.06–1.25) and for thyroid cancer (SIR = 2.39; 95% CI, 1.70–3.27), prostate cancer (SIR = 1.21; 95% CI, 1.01–1.44), combined hematopoietic and lymphoid cancers (SIR = 1.36; 95% CI, 1.07–1.71), and soft tissue cancers (SIR = 2.26; 95% CI, 1.13–4.05). When restricted to 302 cancers diagnosed ≥6 months after enrollment to control for any potential bias from responders enrolling in the program after they become ill, the SIR for all cancers decreased to 1.06 (95% CI, 0.94–1.18), but thyroid and prostate cancer diagnoses remained greater than expected (Table 2). The relative risk of all cancers combined was elevated in the very high-exposure group compared with the low-exposure group (relative risk (RR) = 1.19; 95% CI, 0.70–2.01 in the unrestricted analysis and RR = 1.40; 95% CI, 0.71–2.76 in the restricted analysis). Compared with those who arrived at the WTC sites after 14 September, the incidence of all cancers for the unrestricted analysis was increased in responders who were directly exposed to the dust cloud and in those who experienced significant amounts of dust on 9/11 (RR = 1.22, 95% CI, 0.94–1.58, and RR = 1.32, 95% CI, 1.01–1.73, respectively). The results for the restricted analysis were similar, with an increase in cancer incidence in responders who were directly exposed to the dust cloud (RR = 1.13; 95% CI, 0.79–1.61) and for responders who experienced significant amounts of dust (RR = 1.23; 95% CI, 0.85–1.76).

Table 2 Summary of SIRs for selected cancers from studies of cancer incidence in WTC responders [1, 2, 4]

Cancer site	FDNY; WTC-exposed vs. external referent [1]		FDNY; WTC-exposed vs. internal referent [1]		WTC Health Registry [4]		WTC Consortium unrestricted cohort [2]		WTC Consortium restricted cohort [2]	
	# Obs	SIR (95% CI)	# Obs	SIR (95% CI)	# Obs	SIR (95% CI)	# Obs	SIR (95% CI)	# Obs	SIR (95% CI)
All sites combined	263	1.10(0.98–1.25)	na	1.32(1.07–1.62)	223	1.14(0.99–1.30)	575	1.15(1.06–1.25)	301	1.06(0.94–1.18)
Upper aerodigestive tract										
Lung	9	0.42(0.20–0.86)	na	0.80(0.29–2.18)	13	0.65(0.35–1.12)	43	0.89(0.64–1.20)	18	1.62(0.37–0.98)
Oral cavity and pharynx			na		≤5	0.77(0.25–1.80)	21	1.21(0.75–1.86)	10	1.00(0.48–1.84)
Esophagus	≤5	0.58(0.15–2.32)	na	1.32(0.12–14.5)	≤5	1.16(0.24–3.39)	11	1.67(0.83–2.98)	7	1.77(0.71–3.65)
Stomach	8	2.24(0.98–5.25)	na	1.82(0.44–7.49)	≤5	0.91(0.19–2.67)	11	1.20(0.60–1.26)	7	1.33(0.53–2.74)
Lymphatic and hematologic cancers										
Non-Hodgkin lymphoma	21	1.58(1.03–2.42)	na	1.90(0.87–4.15)	11	1.15(0.57–2.06)	38	1.36(0.96–1.86)	13	0.85(0.45–1.45)
Multiple myeloma	≤5	1.49(0.56–3.97)	na	na	7	2.85(1.15–5.88)	9	1.41(0.64–2.67)	≤5	0.54(N/A)
Leukemia	9	1.40(0.73–2.70)	na	0.98(0.33–2.77)	6	1.25(0.46–2.72)	19	1.41(0.85–2.19)		
Urinary tract										
Urinary bladder	11	1.01(0.56–1.83)	na	1.28(0.47–3.86)	8	0.94(0.41–1.85)	29	1.37(0.92–1.96)	15	1.18(0.66–1.94)
Kidney	10	0.86(0.46–1.60)	na	2.91(0.64–13.3)	12	1.38(0.71–2.41)	31	1.39(0.95–1.98)	17	1.34(0.78–2.14)
Other sites										
Melanoma	33	1.54(1.08–2.18)	na	1.61(0.87–2.99)	10	1.32(0.63–2.43)	20	0.93(0.57–1.43)	12	1.01(0.52–1.77)
Prostate	90	1.49(1.20–1.86)	na	1.11(0.77–1.59)	67	1.43(1.11–1.82)	129	1.21(1.01–1.44)	82	1.23(0.98–1.53)
Thyroid	17	3.07(1.86–5.08)	na	5.21(1.19–22.7)	13	2.02(1.07–3.45)	39	2.39(1.70–3.27)	26	3.12(2.04–4.57)

Stein et al. (2016) conducted a mortality study of 28,918 responders enrolled in the WTCHP between July 16, 2002, and December 31, 2011, who completed examinations at any of six clinical sites consented to participate in research. A total of 16,177 responders was known to be alive due to follow-up visits after the end of 2011, and the remainder ($n = 12,741$) only were linked with the National Death Index (NDI). Social security number (SSN) was available for only 37% of the records sent to NDI for linkage, limiting the quality of the matches. Mortality information from the NDI was supplemented by next-of-kin report. Exposure was categorized as described in the incidence [2] study. Expected numbers of deaths were calculated based on US population rates. Overall mortality in this cohort was significantly decreased (SMR 0.43; 95% CI, 0.39–0.48); an all-cancer SMR was not reported. Most cancer site-specific SMRs were significantly decreased. SMRs for neoplasms of the lymphatic and hematopoietic tissue (SMR = 1.09; 95% CI, 0.66–1.70) and benign and unspecified neoplasms (SMR = 1.15; 95% CI, 0.24–3.36) were slightly, but not significantly, increased.

World Trade Center Registry Enrollees

A cancer incidence study was conducted among enrollees in the World Trade Center (WTC) Health Registry [4]. The WTC Health Registry is an epidemiological cohort study created as a public health response to 9/11. Enrollment in the WTC Health Registry was voluntary for people who lived, worked, or went to school in the area of the WTC disaster, or were involved in rescue and recovery efforts. The registry was open for enrollment in 2003 and 2004, and participants answered a series of questions about where they were on 9/11, their experiences, and their health. Participants were either identified through lists provided by employers, government agencies, and other entities (30%, list identified) or they responded to an outreach campaign (70%, self-identified). Coverage of the eligible population was estimated as 34% for rescue/recovery workers and 23% for residents. A total of 71,434 individuals enrolled in the registry.

The cancer incidence study included registry enrollees who were residents of New York State on 9/11 and had no history of cancer at the time of enrollment [4]. A total of 55,778 individuals were eligible for the study, including 33,928 not involved in rescue/recovery and 21,850 involved in rescue/recovery. The rescue/recovery group included 479 individuals who worked exclusively at the Staten Island recovery operation landfill or on recovery barges. Cancers were identified based on linkage of cohort member records with records of 11 state cancer registries based on the state of residence of the cohort member, and expected numbers of cancers were based on New York State rates. Separate analyses were conducted for rescue/recovery workers and survivors, and separate results were presented for the time period of enrollment through 2006 and 2007 through 2008, with greater emphasis on the results from the latter time period. Among rescue/recovery workers, the SIR for all cancer sites combined in 2007–2008 was not significantly elevated (SIR = 1.14; 95% CI, 0.99–1.30), but SIRs were significantly elevated for three cancer sites: prostate cancer (SIR = 1.43; 95% CI, 1.11–1.82), thyroid cancer (SIR = 2.02; 95% CI, 1.07–3.45), and multiple myeloma (SIR = 2.85; 95% CI, 1.15–5.88). No significantly increased incidence was observed in 2007–2008 among those not involved in rescue/recovery. Hodgkin lymphoma was elevated in the early (SIR = 2.60; 95% CI, 1.12–5.13) but not the later period, and breast cancer was nonsignificantly elevated in both periods (SIR enrollment 2006 = 1.19, 95% CI 0.95–1.48, and SIR 2007–2008 = 1.20, 95% CI, 0.93–1.42). Using within-cohort comparisons, the intensity of World Trade Center exposure was not significantly associated with lung, prostate, and thyroid cancer, non-Hodgkin lymphoma, or hematologic cancer in either group.

A mortality study was also conducted among World Trade Center Registry enrollees [6]. Deaths occurring in 2003–2009 in WTC Health Registry participants residing in New York City were identified through linkage to New York City vital records and the National Death Index. Standardized mortality ratios (SMRs) were calculated with New York City rates from 2000 to 2009 as the reference. Within the cohort, proportional hazards were used to examine the relation between a three-tiered WTC-related exposure level (high, intermediate, or low) and total mortality. A total of 156 deaths were identified in 13,337 rescue and recovery workers and 634 deaths in 28,593 non-rescue and non-recovery participants. All-cause SMRs were significantly lower than that expected for rescue and recovery participants (SMR = 0·45, 95% CI, 0·38–0·53) and non-rescue and non-recovery participants (SMR = 0·61, 95% CI, 0·56–0·66). There were no significantly elevated SMRs for any category of cancer examined.

Police Officers

Cancer incidence was investigated in 39,946 police officers employed by the New York City Police Department on September 11, 2001, followed from 2002 to 2014. The results of this study are difficult to interpret because SIRs were not presented based on an external referent group.

Summary of Findings of Cancer Incidence and Mortality Studies to Date

The results of cancer incidence studies among rescue/recovery workers are summarized in Table 2 and are reviewed below for specific sites.

Cancers of the Upper Aerodigestive Tract

Cancers of the upper aerodigestive tract among WTC responders and survivors are of particular concern for several reasons. The upper aerodigestive tract was a major target organ for non-cancer WTC exposure-related health effects, including chronic nasopharyngitis, upper airway hyperreactivity, chronic laryngitis, interstitial lung disease, "chronic respiratory disorder—fumes/vapors," reactive airway disease syndrome (RADS), and chronic cough syndrome. Inflammatory processes are implicated in many of these conditions and are also considered a mechanism that contributes to cancer development. Cancer of the lung in particular has been associated with a large number of occupational and environmental exposures [7, 12].

Cancer incidence studies in WTC rescue and recovery workers have not detected evidence of an excess in lung cancer incidence (Table 2), which is not surprising for several reasons. The incidence of cancer of the lung in the general population is strongly associated with tobacco smoking. Tobacco smoking prevalence varies dramatically by geographical area, socioeconomic status, occupation, and other factors and has been declining faster in the New York City area than in most other parts of the country due to aggressive tobacco control measures [13–16]. Moreover, rescue and recovery workers who developed WTC-related respiratory conditions may be more likely to stop smoking. Thus, any excess of lung cancer associated with WTC exposure may be difficult to detect using external referent rates, and even internal analyses may need to adjust for differential smoking as well as conduct exposure-response analyses based on estimated intensity and duration of WTC exposure. A second reason why it is not surprising that an excess of lung cancer has not been detected in studies to date is that cancers of the lung resulting from tobacco smoking and from occupational exposures typically take 20 or more years to develop after exposure begins.

Cancers of the oral cavity and pharynx were reported in the World Trade Center Registry cohort and the WTC Consortium cohort with SIRs close to 1.00 (Table 2). Risk factors for cancers of the oral cavity and pharynx in the general population include tobacco smoking, smokeless tobacco, HPV infection, betel quid, and alcohol [7, 12]. The lip, oral cavity, and pharynx are of concern for WTC-exposed rescue and recovery workers because these areas have high potential for direct exposure to toxic materials through hand-to-mouth contact. However, because cancers of the oral cavity and pharynx are strongly related to tobacco use, SIRs based on external referent populations may underestimate the true risk, and it will be important to emphasize internal analyses for these cancers as well.

Slight elevations in the SIRs for cancer of the esophagus were found in the FDNY internal referent analysis and the WTC Registry study, while moderately (but nonsignificantly) increased SIRs were observed in both the unrestricted and restricted cohorts in the WTC Consortium study (Table 2). There are two etiologically distinct subtypes of esophageal cancer, squamous cell, which typically arises in the upper part of the esophagus and is strongly associated with tobacco smoking and alcohol consumption, and adenocarcinoma of the esophagus, which is strongly associated with obesity and gastrointestinal reflux disease (GERD [8]). GERD, a WTC-related health condition, is capable of producing esophageal adenocarcinoma directly or, more commonly, through an intermediate preneoplastic lesion, the Barrett's esophagus (BE). As of June 30, 2016, 16,418 individuals had been certified as having WTC-related GERD by the WTC Health Program. Although treatment of GERD is protective against the development of BE and adenocarcinoma of the esophagus, it will be important to monitor the incidence of esophageal cancer in future updates of the cancer incidence studies among WTC responders and survivors.

Moderate (nonsignificant) elevations in the SIRs for stomach cancer were observed in the FDNY study, small elevations in the WTC Consortium study, and no elevation in the WTC Registry study (Table 2). Since cancer of the distal esophagus, gastroesophageal junction, and gastric cardia share common risk factors, the high prevalence of GERD in WTC rescue and recovery workers suggests that WTC exposures may increase risk of stomach cancer as well.

Lymphatic and Hematologic Cancers

Lymphatic and hematologic cancers are of particular concern among WTC responders and survivors because these cancers have been associated with exposure to a large number of exogenous carcinogens including ionizing radiation, benzene, formaldehyde, reactive chemicals, chemotherapeutic agents, and tobacco smoke [7, 12]. Excess risks of leukemia and lymphomas are often observed after much shorter latency periods than solid tumors. Thus, observation of excess SIRs for these cancers might be seen as an early signal of increased cancer risks associated with WTC exposures. Non-Hodgkin lymphoma (NHL) incidence was moderately elevated in the FDNY cohort, slightly increased in the WTC Registry cohort, and in the unrestricted but not the restricted WTC Consortium study (Table 2). Multiple myeloma, which was the subject of an early case-series report from the WTC Consortium [9], remained moderately elevated in the unrestricted cohort analysis in the cancer incidence study. The SIR for myeloma was substantially elevated in the WTC Registry cohort and moderately elevated in the FDNY study. SIRs > 1.00 were also observed for leukemia in all three studies although none approached statistical significance. The incidence of the lymphatic and hematopoietic cancers will be of great interest in future follow-up of these cohorts.

Cancers of the Urinary Tract

Cancers of the urinary tract are of particular concern because cancer of the bladder in particular has been associated with a variety of exogenous carcinogens, including occupational exposure to carcinogenic aromatic amines, coal tar pitch, and soot as well as tobacco smoking [7, 12]. Most SIRs for bladder and kidney cancer were greater than 1.00 but did not approach statistical significance (Table 2); the highest SIR of 2.91 (CI 0.64–13.3) was reported in the internal referent analysis of the FDNY cohort.

Cancers of Other Sites

The SIR for melanoma was moderately elevated in the FDNY cohort and statistically significant in the external referent analysis, somewhat elevated in the WTC Registry cohort and not elevated in the WTC Consortium study (Table 2). Melanoma has been associated with ultraviolet radiation and polychlorinated biphenyl exposure [7, 12]. Skin examination and biopsy may detect melanoma earlier than they would be detected by patients [10] and therefore increased medical scrutiny in WTC-exposed populations and may play a role in the increased melanoma incidence observed in early follow-up of WTC rescue and recovery workers.

The SIR for prostate cancer was moderately elevated in the FDNY cohort (Table 2) and statistically significant in the external referent analysis. Prostate cancer was statistically significantly elevated in the WTC Registry cohort and the unrestricted analysis of the WTC Consortium cohort (Table 2). Prostate cancer is one of the most common cancers in men and has not been strongly associated with exposure to exogenous carcinogens; there are no agents classified by IARC as having sufficient evidence of causing prostate cancer in humans and only a few classified as having limited evidence [7, 12]. Although prostate cancer has not been strongly associated with exposure to exogenous carcinogens, the etiology of prostate cancer is poorly understood, and therefore it is possible that WTC exposure may have increased prostate cancer risk through the presence of multiple agents or mechanisms unique to the exposure circumstance. The incidence of prostate cancer in the United States has been strongly correlated with the introduction and prevalence of PSA testing [11], and therefore increased healthcare utilization and medical scrutiny may also be a factor in the observed excess in prostate cancer incidence. PSA screening is not offered as part of WTCHP health screening for rescue and recovery workers since the US Preventive Services Task Force recommended against it in 2012 [12].

Thyroid cancer incidence is significantly elevated in all three rescue and recovery worker cohorts (Table 2). There is no recommended screening test for thyroid cancer, but it may be detected as a nodule during a routine medical exam or as an incidental finding in an ultrasound or CT scan of the neck. The incidence of thyroid cancer has been rising rapidly in the United States and many other high-income countries, and most of this increase is thought to be due to increased use of such scans [22]. Exogenous agents associated with thyroid cancer include exposure to radionuclides, including iodine-131 and X and gamma radiation [7, 12].

Summary of Limitations and Strengths of Cancer Incidence and Mortality Studies to Date

An inherent limitation of all of the published studies is the relatively short time of follow-up since 9/11. Excess cancer risks associated with many environmental, occupational, and other exogenous carcinogens (such as tobacco) become apparent only decades after exposure. Thus, it will be extremely important to continue to follow cancer incidence in these populations over time. Population-based registry linkage will facilitate complete and accurate ascertainment of incident cancer cases. Continued follow-up will not only allow for longer latency but also increase the numbers of cancer cases expected based on general population rates, increasing statistical power and ability to conduct exposure-response analyses.

Potential overlap in participation among the various cohorts is of concern, especially since consistency in results for specific cancer sites among the studies will be important in interpreting the results. Overlap between the WTCHP responder cohort and the FDNY cohort is thought to be minimal; however, approximately 20% of responders enrolled in the WTCHP are also registered with the health registry [3].

An important limitation of the WTC Registry and the WTC Consortium studies is the potential biases associated with self-selection into the cohort. This is not a criticism of the methodology of the studies. There was no mechanism to maintain a roster of rescue and recovery workers and others performing paid or volunteer work at the site or residents, students, or individuals employed in the area. The WTC Registry used lists of potentially exposed individuals (such as employees of firms contracted to work at the site and/or located in the area) as well as other forms of outreach for recruiting and obtained a large and fairly representative sample of individuals with various types of exposure. Nonetheless, as in any voluntary study, it is possible that there was differential participation according to socioeconomic status, race/ethnicity, age, or other characteristics. It is also possible that there would have been greater participation among those who felt that they had been affected by WTC exposures or lack of participation among those who were more affected and wished to put the experience behind them. Nonetheless, the registry cohort has been an important source of information on mental and physical health effects in a variety of WTC-exposed populations and will continue to be so for cancer. Moreover, since enrollment in the registry cohort has been closed since 2004, self-selection into the cohort as a result of emerging health conditions after 2004 will not be a concern. The WTC Registry has also been the only source of information about health outcomes of community survivors, including children.

Biases due to self-selection according to health status are an important concern for analysis and interpretation of WTC Consortium studies. Although eligibility for the program is based on WTC-related exposure history and medical monitoring and screening are offered for asymptomatic individuals, it is likely that some members sought care after developing WTC-related symptoms, although not necessarily cancer. Since 2012, many cancers have been designated as WTC-related conditions, and therefore some individuals may have enrolled in the program as a result of their cancer diagnosis. Although various analytic strategies can be employed to address self-selection biases in the WTC Consortium cohort, this will continue to be a challenge as cancer incidence follow-up continues.

The FDNY cohort is the only WTC-exposed rescue and recovery worker cohort that is not affected by self-selection, since it includes all FDNY firefighters employed during a defined time period. An additional strength is the ability to define an internal referent population. Although the statistical power of the study to detect excesses in cancer of specific types is currently limited due to its small size, the statistical power will increase as the cohort ages and the expected numbers of cancers based on general population rates increase.

Conclusion

Although the existing cohorts provide important opportunities to gain knowledge about the cancer risks related to WTC exposures, even after prolonged follow-up, there may be considerable uncertainty about these risks. It's possible that excess cancers could occur in subsets of the populations and not be detectable in epidemiologic studies due to the lack of uniformity of WTC-related exposures and inability to characterize them. The composition of the materials present varied from place to place and day to day, and individual exposures varied according to work activities, proximity to fires, use of respirators and protective clothing, and other factors. If cancer excesses are observed in future follow-up of these cohorts, the variability in exposures and lack of environmental monitoring data may make it difficult to apply criteria for causality such as consistency between studies and evidence of a positive exposure gradient. It is nonetheless important to learn what we can using the best methods we have available. Although we hope to never experience a terrorist attack of this nature and magnitude again, it is important that the public health community be prepared to apply the lessons learned from 9/11 to improve assessment of potential hazards and protection of responders and community residents.

References

1. Zeig-Owens R, Webber MP, Hall CB, Schwartz T, Jaber N, Weakley J, et al. Early assessment of cancer outcomes in new York City firefighters after the 9/11 attacks: an observational cohort study. Lancet. 2011;378(9794):898–905.
2. Solan S, Wallenstein S, Shapiro M, Teitelbaum SL, Stevenson L, Kochman A, et al. Cancer incidence in world trade center rescue and recovery workers, 2001-2008. Environ Health Perspect. 2013;121(6):699–704.
3. Stein CR, Wallenstein S, Shapiro M, Hashim D, Moline JM, Udasin I, et al. Mortality among world trade center rescue and recovery workers, 2002-2011. Am J Ind Med. 2016;59(2):87–95.

4. Li J, Cone JE, Kahn AR, Brackbill RM, Farfel MR, Greene CM, et al. Association between world trade center exposure and excess cancer risk. JAMA. 2012;308(23):2479–88.
5. Jordan HT, Brackbill RM, Cone JE, Debchoudhury I, Farfel MR, Greene CM, et al. Mortality among survivors of the Sept 11, 2001, world trade center disaster: results from the world trade center health registry cohort. Lancet. 2011;378(9794):879–87.
6. Woskie SR, Kim H, Freund A, Stevenson L, Park BY, Baron S, et al. World trade center disaster: assessment of responder occupations, work locations, and job tasks. Am J Ind Med. 2011;54(9):681–95.
7. List of Classifications by cancer sites with *sufficient* or *limited* evidence in humans, Volumes 1 to 116; adapted from Table 4 in Cogliano et al. 2011. 201. Available from: https://monographs.iarc.fr/ENG/Classification/Table4.pdf
8. Domper Arnal MJ, Ferrandez Arenas A, Lanas Arbeloa A. Esophageal cancer: risk factors, screening and endoscopic treatment in western and eastern countries. World J Gastroenterol. 2015;21(26):7933–43.
9. Moline JM, Herbert R, Crowley L, Troy K, Hodgman E, Shukla G, et al. Multiple myeloma in world trade center responders: a case series. J Occup Environ Med. 2009;51(8):896–902.
10. Welch HG, Woloshin S, Schwartz LM. Skin biopsy rates and incidence of melanoma: population based ecological study. BMJ. 2005;331(7515):481.
11. Jemal A, Fedewa SA, Ma J, Siegel R, Lin CC, Brawley O, et al. Prostate cancer incidence and PSA testing patterns in relation to USPSTF screening recommendations. JAMA. 2015;314(19):2054–61.
12. Moyer VA, Force USPST. Screening for prostate cancer: U.S. preventive services task Force recommendation statement. Ann Intern Med. 2012;157(2):120–34.
13. Aldrich TK, Gustave J, Hall CB, Cohen HW, Webber MP, Zeig-Owens R, et al. Lung function in rescue workers at the world trade center after 7 years. N Engl J Med. 2010;362(14):1263–72.
14. Kleinman EJ, Christos PJ, Gerber LM, Reilly JP, Moran WF, Einstein AJ, et al. NYPD cancer incidence rates 1995–2014 encompassing the entire world trade center cohort. J Occup Environ Med. 2015;57(10):e101–13.
15. Boffetta P, Zeig-Owens R, Wallenstein S, Li J, Brackbill R, Cone J, et al. Cancer in world trade center responders: findings from multiple cohorts and options for future study. Am J Ind Med. 2016;59(2):96–105.
16. Wisnivesky JP, Teitelbaum SL, Todd AC, Boffetta P, Crane M, Crowley L, et al. Persistence of multiple illnesses in world trade center rescue and recovery workers: a cohort study. Lancet. 2011;378(9794):888–97.
17. Cogliano VJ, Baan R, Straif K, Grosse Y, Lauby-Secretan B, El Ghissassi F, et al. Preventable exposures associated with human cancers. J Natl Cancer Inst. 2011;103(24):1827–39.
18. Islami F, Ward EM, Jacobs EJ, Ma J, Goding Sauer A, Lortet-Tieulent J, et al. Potentially preventable premature lung cancer deaths in the USA if overall population rates were reduced to those of educated whites in lower-risk states. Cancer Causes Control. 2015;26(3):409–18.
19. Jamal A, Homa DM, O'Connor E, Babb SD, Caraballo RS, Singh T, et al. Current cigarette smoking among adults–United States, 2005–2014. MMWR Morb Mortal Wkly Rep. 2015;64(44):1233–40.
20. Kilgore EA, Mandel-Ricci J, Johns M, Coady MH, Perl SB, Goodman A, et al. Making it harder to smoke and easier to quit: the effect of 10 years of tobacco control in new York City. Am J Public Health. 2014;104(6):e5–8.
21. Syamlal G, Mazurek JM, Hendricks SA, Jamal A. Cigarette smoking trends among U.S. working adult by industry and occupation: findings from the 2004–2012 National Health Interview Survey. Nicotine Tob Res. 2015;17(5):599–606.
22. Davies L, Welch HG. Increasing incidence of thyroid cancer in the United States, 1973–2002. JAMA. 2006;295(18):2164–7.
23. Lioy PJ, Weisel CP, Millette JR, Eisenreich S, Vallero D, Offenberg J, et al. Characterization of the dust/smoke aerosol that settled east of the world trade center (WTC) in lower Manhattan after the collapse of the WTC 11 September 2001. Environ Health Perspect. 2002;110(7):703–14.

World Trade Center Asthma

Alpa G. Desai and Gwen S. Skloot

Introduction

More than 40,000 men and women were exposed to products of combustion and particulate matter as a result of the terrorist attacks on the World Trade Center (WTC) on September 11, 2001 [1]. Pulverization of the structural components of the towers released a plume of dust and ash into lower Manhattan and beyond. The dust was a complex mixture of over 400 substances including glass fibers, asbestos, silica, lead, polycyclic aromatic hydrocarbons, metals, and polychlorinated biphenyls [2] with a particulate matter concentration of 100,000 mg/m [3]. In addition, prolonged smoldering fires [4] emitted gaseous and particulate combustion products. Exposures were ongoing for hundreds of thousands of people who lived, worked, or volunteered in the area since recovery and cleanup efforts took 9.5 months to complete [4]. Multiple studies have reported increased rates of asthma as well as worsening of preexisting asthma in those exposed [4–9]. Although most of the particulate matter was expected to deposit in the upper airway, it is clear that lower airway deposition and injury occurred. Longitudinal studies have demonstrated persistent airway hyperresponsiveness (AHR) years after the attacks. This chapter discusses the following aspects of WTC asthma: epidemiology, pathogenesis and risk factors, clinical presentation and comorbidities of disease, as well as a multidisciplinary approach to management.

A.G. Desai
Division of Pulmonary, Critical Care and Sleep Medicine, HSC 17-040, Stony Brook University, Stony Brook, NY 11794-8172, USA
e-mail: alpa.desai@stonybrookmedicine.edu

G.S. Skloot (✉)
Division of Pulmonary, Critical Care and Sleep Medicine, Icahn School of Medicine at Mount Sinai, Box #1232, One Gustave L. Levy Place, New York, NY 10029, USA
e-mail: gwen.skloot@mssm.edu

© Springer International Publishing AG 2018　　　　　　　　　　　　　　　　95
A.M. Szema (ed.), *World Trade Center Pulmonary Diseases and Multi-Organ System Manifestations*, DOI 10.1007/978-3-319-59372-2_7

WTC Asthma Epidemiology

It is difficult to clearly define the scope of WTC asthma prevalence. Symptom-based surveys have identified increased incidence of self-reported asthma for 18 months following the attack [10]. A WTC registry of rescue and recovery workers ($n = 25,748$) documented self-reported post-9/11 asthma in 926 workers for a 3-year incidence rate of 3.6%, or 12 times higher than that expected for the general adult population [11]. Increased incidence of new-onset asthma has been associated with the time of arrival at the site, cumulative exposure, and lack of appropriate respiratory protections [12]. Twenty seven percent of New York City residents reported increased asthma symptoms in the weeks after the disaster [13] although it is not clear how many of these individuals had pre-existing asthma.

Pathogenesis

WTC asthma is a distinct entity that arose in individuals exposed to products of combustion and particulate matter following the collapse of the towers on 9/11. Although most of the particulate matter (>90%) was >10 μm [2] and expected to deposit mainly in the upper airways, mouth breathing and alkalinity of the material impaired nasal clearance. Analyzed samples were highly alkaline, with a pH > 10. WTC responders breathed at high minute ventilations where mouth breathing predominates [6]. Though only a small percentage of particles were <10 μm (i.e., respirable fraction), the enormity of the dust cloud still led to significant exposure for many individuals. Induced sputum testing in a sample of highly exposed NYC firefighters has demonstrated WTC dust in the lower airways measuring >10 μm [14].

WTC asthma is part of the spectrum of disorders ranging from reactive airways dysfunction syndrome (RADS) that involves an acute high-level irritant exposure to irritant-induced asthma with recurrent lower-level exposures [5, 6, 15]. The mechanism of injury is believed to be non-immunologic [16, 17]. Asthma symptoms are due to direct airway epithelial damage with release of pro-inflammatory mediators [18]. Pathologic changes of the airways include denuded epithelium, submucosal chronic inflammation, and focal thickening of the basement membrane [19]. The inflammatory process of irritant-induced asthma is not thought to be primarily Th2 cell mediated [20]. In a mouse model, acute exposure to high levels of WTC particulate matter induced mild pulmonary neutrophilic inflammation and marked AHR to inhaled methacholine [21]. Interestingly, Kazeros et al. reported peripheral eosinophilia that correlated with persistent wheeze and airflow obstruction in WTC disaster-exposed residents and workers [22]. Although eosinophilia is generally thought typical of Th2-related inflammation, asthma is phenotypically heterogeneous, and a "low Th2" lymphocyte/eosinophil cohort has been described based on analysis of bronchial epithelial cells [22, 23]. Induced sputum analysis in a study of 39 WTC firefighters revealed rising neutrophil and eosinophil counts with increasing work duration [14]. In the same study, sputum analysis also revealed elevated metalloproteinases (MMP)-9 levels in WTC firefighters [14]. Metalloproteinases (MMPs) are also thought to play a role in the airway remodeling of asthma and in the induction of AHR [24].

Nolan et al. [3] demonstrated that elevated granulocyte-macrophage colony-stimulating factor (GM-CSF) and macrophage-derived chemokine (MDC) were associated with subsequent increased risk of airflow obstruction in WTC disaster-exposed firefighters with normal pre-September 11, 2001, forced expiratory volume in 1 s (FEV_1), suggesting that such inflammatory biomarkers were important in the pathogenesis of asthma post-9/11. Others have shown that human bronchial epithelial cell produce GM-CSF in response to particulate matter [25, 26] and that MDC is elevated in the bronchoalveolar lavage fluid of asthmatic patients. Different WTC-related exposures and individual susceptibility to exposure (lower baseline lung function) may have influenced the levels of these biomarkers and their physiologic impact.

Regardless of the predominant inflammatory cellular subtype and the cytokine milieu, the consequences of allergic asthma and irritant-induced asthma are the same with AHR and airflow obstruction with or without reversibility [16, 17]. It is possible that WTC asthma is phenotypically heterogeneous although this is not yet known.

Risk Factors

Risk factors for the development of WTC asthma relate predominantly to the magnitude of irritant exposure.

A clear exposure-response gradient exists, with most severe asthma symptoms in those directly exposed to the dust cloud on the morning of 9/11 [27–29]. In a prospective cohort study, airway hyperreactivity at 1, 3, and 6 months was associated with exposure intensity (evaluated by self-administered questionnaires), independent of ex-smoking and airflow obstruction [27]. At 6 months after collapse of the towers, highly exposed workers (on site on the morning of day 1) were 6.8× more likely than moderately exposed workers (arrived on the afternoon of day 1 or during day 2) and controls (workers absent from the site during the first 2 weeks or longer) to be hyperactive [27]. Each additional month of work increased the likelihood of respiratory symptoms by 8–11% [30], although the effect on new-onset asthma is not specifically known.

Risk factors associated with an increased incidence of WTC asthma are shown in Table 1. Among WTC workers who arrived at the disaster site on 9/11/01, increased time to mask or respirator use was associated with a greater risk for the development of asthma [11]. In one study of 1660 individuals with high-intensity exposure (arriving on the morning of the collapse of the towers) at the WTC site, only 22% of workers reported frequent mask use [31]. In another study, respirators were worn rarely or not at all by 93% on the day of the collapse, 85% on the day after, and 76%

Table 1 Risk factor for WTC asthma

Increased incidence of WTC asthma associated with:
Dust cloud exposure on the morning of 9/11
Earlier arrival time relative to collapse
Work on the "pile"
Cumulative exposure (particularly >90 days)

Adapted from [11]

on the second through sixth days after the attack [29]. There were multiple reasons for lack of respirator use including lack of adherence and availability of masks for many responders [31].

In some reports, the workers' role at the site was a risk factor for new-onset asthma. This was particularly true for firefighters, who had heavier dust exposures than other workers. The significance of these reports was enhanced by the availability of lung function and methacholine bronchoprovocation data that preceded the exposure [8, 31]. Although there are many reports of respiratory symptoms in multiple other rescue/recovery workers, volunteers, lower Manhattan residents, and office workers, these do not specifically link the symptoms to new-onset asthma [31–34].

Smoking status was an additive risk factor for WTC asthma [5]. Other reports on irritant-induced asthma demonstrate that tobacco use at the time of inhalational resulted in lower FEV_1 and FEV_1/FVC, as well as in increased AHR [5, 18, 35, 36].

Preexisting atopy can predispose individuals to develop irritant-induced asthma in general [18], though this was not clearly demonstrated in the WTC population [37]. In fact, the atopy prevalence in this WTC population was similar to that of the general US population [37].

Age may have also influenced the risk of new onset asthma in those with WTC exposure, but data on this are limited.

Clinical Presentation

Upper and lower respiratory symptoms were common in individuals exposed at the WTC disaster [4–7, 28, 29, 38, 39]. In most cases, the onset of symptoms consistent with asthma began within 6 months following irritant exposure at the WTC site [5]. Individuals diagnosed with WTC asthma presented similarly to the general asthma patient with chest tightness, exertional and non-exertional dyspnea, wheezing, and cough [29]. Diurnal variation of symptoms and sensitivity to fumes, weather extremes, and other classic asthma triggers are common. Patients typically complain of nighttime awakenings with asthma that is not ideally controlled. One unique clinical feature of this population was the "WTC cough," described as persistent cough syndrome recurring during the 6 months after 9/11. WTC cough was associated with underlying airway inflammation and symptoms of rhinosinusitis, bronchitis, and GERD [29]. Workers with preexisting asthma may have experienced greater severity of asthma symptoms than controls [7].

Multiple studies have evaluated lung function in those exposed at the WTC disaster, but not all of these individuals carry the diagnosis of asthma [1, 3, 28, 31, 40, 41]. Although an obstructive pattern is described, other studies have reported a restrictive pattern with or without air trapping [40]. In the setting of small airway obstruction, forced expiratory maneuvers may result in bronchial collapse and cessation of airflow. The airways that close off at a higher than normal closing volume during the maneuver do not contribute to the full vital capacity or to FEV_1 after closing volume is reached, resulting in a proportional drop in forced vital capacity (FVC) and FEV_1 [42]. This allows for a maintained FEV_1/FVC ratio and explains the restrictive pattern [43, 44].

AHR and variable response to bronchodilator has also been demonstrated [1, 8, 27, 29]. In fact, Banauch et al. found that AHR developing shortly after the WTC attacks predicted RADS at 6 months in highly exposed workers (present within 2 h of the towers' collapse) [27] (Fig. 1).

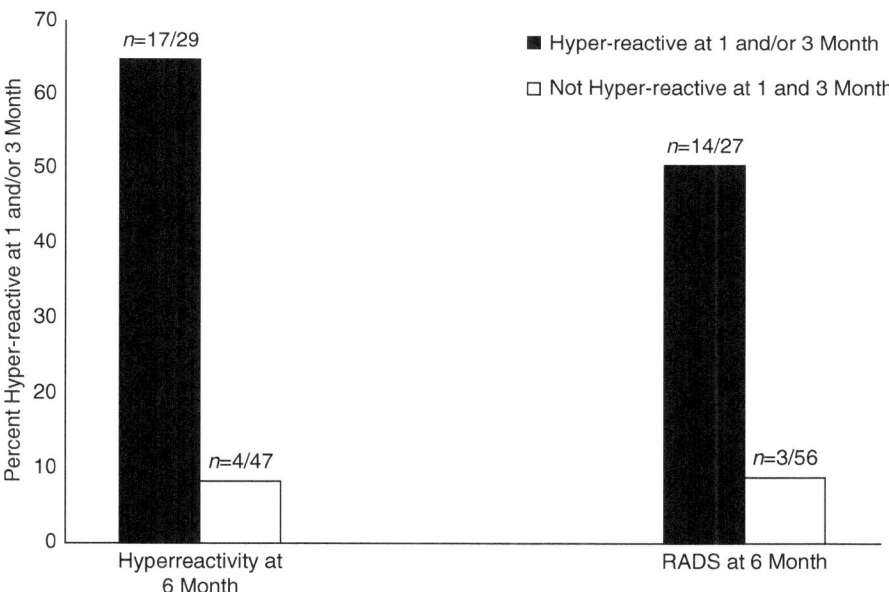

Fig. 1 Highly exposed subjects who were hyper-reactive at 1 or at 3 months were more often hyper-reactive at 6 months. Highly exposed subjects who were hyper-reactive at 1 or at 3 months had RADS (defined as both symptomatic and hyper-reactive) at 6 months significantly more often ($p = 0.021$) than those who were not hyper-reactive. Reprinted with permission of the American Thoracic Society. Copyright © 2017 American Thoracic Society [27]. The American Journal of Respiratory and Critical Care Medicine is an official journal of the American Thoracic Society

Interestingly, many individuals had normal spirometry despite significant respiratory symptoms, which may point to a lack of sensitivity of spirometry to fully demonstrate abnormalities of airway function [28, 45]. In a study of ironworkers exposed at the WTC disaster, lung function abnormalities were far more evident by forced oscillometry (FO) testing than by spirometry [28]. Similarly, while spirometric response to bronchodilator was variable, there was a higher prevalence of bronchodilator response as assessed by FO [28, 46]. FO has shown correlation between asthma symptoms and isolated small airways dysfunction even in the setting of normal spirometry [47]. FO evidence of small airway disease, possibly at the level of the terminal bronchiole, has been an important finding and may be a key characteristic of asthma in the WTC population [28, 46, 48].

Chest imaging is not typically used to diagnose asthma (unless utilized to exclude other entities), but it has played a larger role in WTC patients and has been correlated with physiologic data. Inspiratory and expiratory chest CT findings may demonstrate air trapping and bronchial wall thickening [49, 50]. Though not diagnostic, this may help support a diagnosis of asthma in cases where clinical symptoms are consistent.

Comorbidities

Comorbidities that impacted the presentation of asthma were common in those exposed at the WTC disaster. There was an increased prevalence of chronic rhinosinusitis in those with highest WTC dust exposure (reactive upper airway dysfunction syndrome (RUDS)) [6]. One study of 1138 rescue/recovery workers and volunteers found 92% had new or worsened ear, nose, and throat symptoms [11], including nasal congestion/drip, sore throat, and sinusitis.

Gastroesophageal reflux disease was found in up to 45% of FDNY rescue workers between 1 and 6 months after collapse, with higher rates in those with bronchial hyper-reactivity [27]. Also, in a survey of 332 firefighters with WTC cough, 87% reported heartburn, often with findings of laryngopharyngeal reflux disease [5, 29]. GERD was associated with spirometric abnormalities and with a diagnosis of WTC-related lower airway disease [51]. It is unclear if GERD is a cause, effect, or complication of asthma, but concurrent treatment is essential to optimize asthma control.

Increasing WTC exposure was associated with a trend toward more severe obstructive sleep apnea (OSA) [52], although further studies are necessary to confirm this association. Additionally, a significant relationship exists between OSA and poorly and very poorly controlled asthma [53]. Treating OSA can improve asthma symptoms in individuals with concurrent OSA [54] although we are not aware of any studies demonstrating this in WTC patients.

COPD was also seen in those exposed at the WTC disaster. This is particularly important since individuals may have the asthma-COPD overlap syndrome.

Extensive review of available literature did not reveal any data in the WTC population, but this is a particularly challenging comorbidity as irreversible airway obstruction can make treatment less effective. It was suspected when fixed obstruction, hyperinflation, decreased diffusion capacity, and/or emphysematous changes on CT were present in individuals who smoked cigarettes [5].

Post-traumatic stress disorder (PTSD) was experienced by many who were exposed to the WTC attacks. PTSD may considerably impact the individual's as well as the healthcare worker's perception of respiratory symptoms, thereby delaying or confounding the diagnosis of asthma and treatment [10, 53].

Diagnostic Evaluation of WTC Asthma

As with traditional asthma, the diagnosis of WTC-related asthma should be suspected in patients with typical respiratory symptoms provoked by classic triggers. Differential diagnosis includes chronic obstructive pulmonary disease (COPD), bronchitis, bronchiectasis, bronchiolitis, hyperventilation/panic attacks, chronic sinusitis, GERD, vocal cord dysfunction, recurrent respiratory infections, and heart disease [55]. It is important to assess for comorbidities that can worsen asthma symptoms, contribute to the pathophysiology of the disease, and influence treatment response [56].

Clinical evaluation should include a focused history and physical exam, detailed assessment of clinical symptoms, occupation and WTC-related exposure history (e.g., arrival time, exposure time, work performed, and use of respirator) (Fig. 2).

Diagnostic challenges in this population include the fact that (1) multiple comorbidities may impact the presentation, (2) the spirometric pattern may not be typical for asthma (i.e., restrictive pattern or isolated small airways dysfunction) [5, 28, 40, 46], and (3) bronchial hyper-reactivity may be intermittent or disappear in irritant-induced asthma with time after exposure removal [4, 57].

Treatment of WTC-related asthma should follow the same guidelines for asthma patients in general [54, 58]. Inhaled corticosteroid therapy is the cornerstone of asthma therapy for symptom control. Short-acting beta agonists are used as rescue medications. Importantly, treatment of WTC asthma patients involves limiting irritant exposure and addressing the multiple physical and mental health comorbidities that often coexist and can decrease asthma control. There is a dose-response relationship with the number of mental health conditions (PTSD, depression, and generalized anxiety disorder) and poorer asthma control [53]. Specialists from allergy and immunology, gastroenterology, otolaryngology, occupational and environmental medicine, and psychiatry must work together with pulmonologists and primary care practitioners to manage WTC-related asthma. Various multidisciplinary treatment centers exist in the tri-state area and function in such a capacity to provide individualized diagnostic and management services to this population.

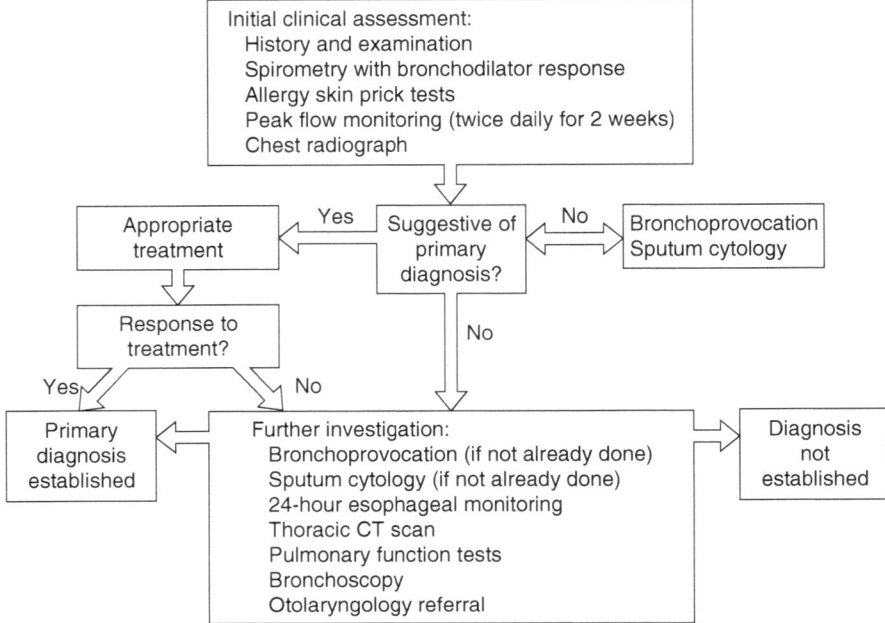

Fig. 2 Algorithm for the diagnostic evaluation of lower respiratory symptoms among former World Trade Center workers and volunteers [4]

Longitudinal Follow-Up and Prognosis of WTC Asthma

There have been multiple studies demonstrating decline in lung function in individuals exposed to WTC dust [1, 12, 31, 48]. Skloot et al. found high rates of abnormal spirometric indices (particularly a low FVC) among non-FDNY workers [1]. Although the majority of the cohort manifested normal decline of lung function between baseline and follow-up (about 3 years later), a small percentage were rapid decliners, losing >300 mL/year of FVC [1]. Aldrich et al. also discovered initially decreased FEV_1 values in its firefighter and EMS workers, with ongoing lung function decline from 2002 to 2008 [12]. The firefighters had an average decline in FEV_1 of 600 mL during this 6-year period [12]. In individuals with persistent lung function decline, it is possible that airway inflammation may progress to remodeling [12]. This may also explain why AHR can continue after termination of exposure in spite of appropriate therapy [8].

Since many responders were previously healthy and fit, a greater loss of function may be required before pulmonary function tests appear abnormal. For those workers without pre-9/11 spirometric data, identifying and treating asthma may be particularly challenging.

In conclusion, asthma continues to be a significant problem in individuals exposed to particulate matter as a result of the WTC disaster. Although some have improved, others have persistent and often difficult-to-control lower respiratory symptoms. The impact of comorbidities on WTC asthma is substantial. As the WTC-exposed population ages, the structural and functional changes of the lung associated with normal aging (i.e., mechanical changes resulting in decreased airway caliber and decreased airflow) may lead to more severe asthma in those affected. Since the trajectory of lung function decline in WTC asthma over many years is not yet known, continued long-term monitoring is imperative to effectively evaluate and manage this population.

References

1. Skloot GS, Schechter CB, Herbert R, Moline JM, Levin SM, Crowley LE, et al. Longitudinal assessment of spirometry in the World Trade Center medical monitoring program. Chest. 2009;135(2):492–8.
2. Lioy PJ, Weisel CP, Millette JR, Eisenreich S, Vallero D, Offenberg J, et al. Characterization of the dust/smoke aerosol that settled east of the World Trade Center (WTC) in lower Manhattan after the collapse of the WTC 11 September 2001. Environ Health Perspect. 2002;110(7):703–14.
3. Nolan A, Naveed B, Comfort AL, Ferrier N, Hall CB, Kwon S, et al. Inflammatory biomarkers predict airflow obstruction after exposure to World Trade Center dust. Chest. 2012;142(2):412–8.
4. de la Hoz RE. Occupational asthma and lower airway disease among World Trade Center workers and volunteers. Curr Allergy Asthma Rep. 2010;10(4):287–94.
5. de la Hoz RE, Shohet MR, Chasan R, Bienenfeld LA, Afilaka AA, Levin SM, et al. Occupational toxicant inhalation injury: the World Trade Center (WTC) experience. Int Arch Occup Environ Health. 2008;81(4):479–85.
6. Prezant DJ, Levin S, Kelly KJ, Aldrich TK. Upper and lower respiratory diseases after occupational and environmental disasters. Mt Sinai J Med. 2008;75(2):89–100.
7. Mauer MP, Cummings KR, Hoen R. Long-term respiratory symptoms in World Trade Center responders. Occup Med. 2010;60(2):145–51.
8. Banauch GI, Dhala A, Alleyne D, Alva R, Santhyadka G, Krasko A, et al. Bronchial hyperreactivity and other inhalation lung injuries in rescue/recovery workers after the World Trade Center collapse. Crit Care Med. 2005;33(1 Suppl):S102–6.
9. Herbert R, Moline J, Skloot G, Metzger K, Baron S, Luft B, et al. The World Trade Center disaster and the health of workers: five-year assessment of a unique medical screening program. Environ Health Perspect. 2006;114(12):1853–8.
10. Brackbill RM, Hadler JL, DiGrande L, Ekenga CC, Farfel MR, Friedman S, et al. Asthma and posttraumatic stress symptoms 5 to 6 years following exposure to the World Trade Center terrorist attack. JAMA. 2009;302(5):502–16.
11. Wheeler K, McKelvey W, Thorpe L, Perrin M, Cone J, Kass D, et al. Asthma diagnosed after 11 September 2001 among rescue and recovery workers: findings from the World Trade Center Health Registry. Environ Health Perspect. 2007;115(11):1584–90.
12. Aldrich TK, Gustave J, Hall CB, Cohen HW, Webber MP, Zeig-Owens R, et al. Lung function in rescue workers at the World Trade Center after 7 years. N Engl J Med. 2010;362(14):1263–72.

13. From the Centers for Disease Control and Prevention. Self-reported increase in asthma severity after the September 11 attacks on the World Trade Center--Manhattan, New York, 2001. JAMA. 2002;288(12):1466–7.

14. Fireman EM, Lerman Y, Ganor E, Greif J, Fireman-Shoresh S, Lioy PJ, et al. Induced sputum assessment in New York City firefighters exposed to World Trade Center dust. Environ Health Perspect. 2004;112(15):1564–9.

15. Mayer A, Pacheco K. RADS and its variants: asthma by another name. Immunol Allergy Clin North Am. 2013;33(1):79–93.

16. Brooks SM, Weiss MA, Bernstein IL. Reactive airways dysfunction syndrome (RADS). Persistent asthma syndrome after high level irritant exposures. Chest. 1985;88(3):376–84.

17. Vandenplas O, Wiszniewska M, Raulf M, de Blay F, Gerth van Wijk R, Moscato G, et al. EAACI position paper: irritant-induced asthma. Allergy. 2014;69(9):1141–53.

18. Quirce S, Gala G, Perez-Camo I, Sanchez-Fernandez C, Pacheco A, Losada E. Irritant-induced asthma: clinical and functional aspects. J Asthma. 2000;37(3):267–74.

19. Bernstein IL, Bernstein DI. Reactive airways disease syndrome RADS after exposure to toxic ammonia fumes. J Allergy Clin Immunol. 1989;83(1):173–9.

20. Chang-Yeung M, Lam S, Kennedy SM, Frew AJ. Persistent asthma after repeated exposure to high concentrations of gases in pulpmills. Am J Respir Crit Care Med. 1994;149(6):1676–80.

21. Gavett SH, Haykal-Coates N, Highfill JW, Ledbetter AD, Chen LC, Cohen MD, et al. World Trade Center fine particulate matter causes respiratory tract hyperresponsiveness in mice. Environ Health Perspect. 2003;111(7):981–91.

22. Kazeros A, Maa MT, Patrawalla P, Liu M, Shao Y, Qian M, et al. Elevated peripheral eosinophils are associated with new-onset and persistent wheeze and airflow obstruction in world trade center-exposed individuals. J Asthma. 2013;50(1):25–32.

23. Woodruff PG, Modrek B, Choy DF, Jia G, Abbas AR, Ellwanger A, et al. T-helper type 2-driven inflammation defines major subphenotypes of asthma. Am J Respir Crit Care Med. 2009;180(5):388–95.

24. Kumagai K, Ohno I, Okada S, Ohkawara Y, Suzuki K, Shinya T, et al. Inhibition of matrix metalloproteinases prevents allergen-induced airway inflammation in a murine model of asthma. J Immunol. 1999;162(7):4212–9.

25. Liu L, Jarjour NN, Busse WW, Kelly EA. Enhanced generation of helper T type 1 and 2 chemokines in allergen-induced asthma. Am J Respir Crit Care Med. 2004;169(10):1118–24.

26. Reibman J, Hsu Y, Chen LC, Kumar A, WC S, Choy W, et al. Size fractions of ambient particulate matter induce granulocyte macrophage colony-stimulating factor in human bronchial epithelial cells by mitogen-activated protein kinase pathways. Am J Respir Cell Mol Biol. 2002;27(4):455–62.

27. Banauch GI, Alleyne D, Sanchez R, Olender K, Cohen HW, Weiden M, et al. Persistent hyperreactivity and reactive airway dysfunction in firefighters at the World Trade Center. Am J Respir Crit Care Med. 2003;168(1):54–62.

28. Skloot G, Goldman M, Fischler D, Goldman C, Schechter C, Levin S, et al. Respiratory symptoms and physiologic assessment of ironworkers at the World Trade Center disaster site. Chest. 2004;125(4):1248–55.

29. Prezant DJ, Weiden M, Banauch GI, McGuinness G, Rom WN, Aldrich TK, et al. Cough and bronchial responsiveness in firefighters at the World Trade Center site. N Engl J Med. 2002;347(11):806–15.

30. Webber MP, Gustave J, Lee R, Niles JK, Kelly K, Cohen HW, et al. Trends in respiratory symptoms of firefighters exposed to the world trade center disaster: 2001-2005. Environ Health Perspect. 2009;117(6):975–80.

31. Banauch GI, Hall C, Weiden M, Cohen HW, Aldrich TK, Christodoulou V, et al. Pulmonary function after exposure to the World Trade Center collapse in the New York City Fire Department. Am J Respir Crit Care Med. 2006;174(3):312–9.

32. Feldman DM, Baron SL, Bernard BP, Lushniak BD, Banauch G, Arcentales N, et al. Symptoms, respirator use, and pulmonary function changes among New York City firefighters responding to the World Trade Center disaster. Chest. 2004;125(4):1256–64.
33. Tao XG, Massa J, Ashwell L, Davis K, Schwab M, Geyh A. The world trade center clean up and recovery worker cohort study: respiratory health amongst cleanup workers approximately 20 months after initial exposure at the disaster site. J Occup Environ Med. 2007;49(10):1063–72.
34. Debchoudhury I, Welch AE, Fairclough MA, Cone JE, Brackbill RM, Stellman SD, et al. Comparison of health outcomes among affiliated and lay disaster volunteers enrolled in the World Trade Center Health Registry. Prev Med. 2011;53(6):359–63.
35. Gautrin D, Leroyer C, Infante-Rivard C, Ghezzo H, Dufour JG, Girard D, et al. Longitudinal assessment of airway caliber and responsiveness in workers exposed to chlorine. Am J Respir Crit Care Med. 1999;160(4):1232–7.
36. Malo JL, L'Archeveque J, Castellanos L, Lavoie K, Ghezzo H, Maghni K. Long-term outcomes of acute irritant-induced asthma. Am J Respir Crit Care Med. 2009;179(10):923–8.
37. de la Hoz RE, Shohet MR, Wisnivesky JP, Bienenfeld LA, Afilaka AA, Herbert R. Atopy and upper and lower airway disease among former World Trade Center workers and volunteers. J Occup Environ Med. 2009;51(9):992–5.
38. de la Hoz RE. Occupational lower airway disease in relation to World Trade Center inhalation exposure. Curr Opin Allergy Clin Immunol. 2011;11(2):97–102.
39. Mauer MP, Herdt-Losavio ML, Carlson GA. Asthma and lower respiratory symptoms in New York State employees who responded to the World Trade Center disaster. Int Arch Occup Environ Health. 2010;83(1):21–7.
40. Berger KI, Reibman J, Oppenheimer BW, Vlahos I, Harrison D, Goldring RM. Lessons from the World Trade Center disaster: airway disease presenting as restrictive dysfunction. Chest. 2013;144(1):249–57.
41. Rom WN, Reibman J, Rogers L, Weiden MD, Oppenheimer B, Berger K, et al. Emerging exposures and respiratory health: world Trade Center dust. Proc Am Thorac Soc. 2010;7(2):142–5.
42. Howard P. The airway as starling resistor. Bull Physiopathol Respir. 1971;7(2):467–74.
43. Hudgel DW, Cooper D, Souhrada J. Reversible restrictive lung disease stimulating asthma. Ann Intern Med. 1976;85(3):328–32.
44. Miller A, Palecki A. Restrictive impairment in patients with asthma. Respir Med. 2007; 101(2):272–6.
45. Salzman SH, Moosavy FM, Miskoff JA, Friedmann P, Fried G, Rosen MJ. Early respiratory abnormalities in emergency services police officers at the World Trade Center site. J Occup Environ Med. 2004;46(2):113–22.
46. Oppenheimer BW, Goldring RM, Herberg ME, Hofer IS, Reyfman PA, Liautaud S, et al. Distal airway function in symptomatic subjects with normal spirometry following World Trade Center dust exposure. Chest. 2007;132(4):1275–82.
47. Berger K, Turetz M, Liu M, Shao Y, Kazeros A, Parsia S, Caplan-Shaw C, Friedman SM, Maslow CB, Marmor M, Goldring RM, Reibman J. Oscillometry complements spirometry in evaluation of subjects following toxic inhalation. ERJ Open Res. 2015;1(2):1–10.
48. Guidotti TL, Prezant D, de la Hoz RE, Miller A. The evolving spectrum of pulmonary disease in responders to the World Trade Center tragedy. Am J Ind Med. 2011;54(9):649–60.
49. Mendelson DS, Roggeveen M, Levin SM, Herbert R, de la Hoz RE. Air trapping detected on end-expiratory high-resolution computed tomography in symptomatic World Trade Center rescue and recovery workers. J Occup Environ Med. 2007;49(8):840–5.
50. Weiden MD, Ferrier N, Nolan A, Rom WN, Comfort A, Gustave J, et al. Obstructive airways disease with air trapping among firefighters exposed to World Trade Center dust. Chest. 2010;137(3):566–74.
51. de la Hoz RE, Christie J, Teamer JA, Bienenfeld LA, Afilaka AA, Crane M, et al. Reflux symptoms and disorders and pulmonary disease in former World Trade Center rescue and recovery workers and volunteers. J Occup Environ Med. 2008;50(12):1351–4.

52. de la Hoz RE, Aurora RN, Landsbergis P, Bienenfeld LA, Afilaka AA, Herbert R. Snoring and obstructive sleep apnea among former World Trade Center rescue workers and volunteers. J Occup Environ Med. 2010;52(1):29–32.
53. Jordan HT, Stellman SD, Reibman J, Farfel MR, Brackbill RM, Friedman SM, et al. Factors associated with poor control of 9/11-related asthma 10-11 years after the 2001 World Trade Center terrorist attacks. J Asthma. 2015;52(6):630–7.
54. National Heart LaBI. Expert Panel report 3: guidelines for the diagnosis and management of asthma. National Institutes of Health. Report No. 07-4051. 28 Aug 2007.
55. Chung KF, Wenzel SE, Brozek JL, Bush A, Castro M, Sterk PJ, et al. International ERS/ATS guidelines on definition, evaluation and treatment of severe asthma. Eur Respir J. 2014;43(2):343–73.
56. Kaplan AG, Balter MS, Bell AD, Kim H, McIvor RA. Diagnosis of asthma in adults. CMAJ. 2009;181(10):E210–20.
57. Malo JL, Ghezzo H. Recovery of methacholine responsiveness after end of exposure in occupational asthma. Am J Respir Crit Care Med. 2004;169(12):1304–7.
58. (GINA) GIfA. Global strategy for asthma management and prevention. 2016.

World Trade Center Dust: Composition and Spatial-Temporal Considerations for Health

Marc Kostrubiak

Introduction

On September 11, 2001, 1.2 million tons of dust and debris were released onto one of the most densely populated areas in the country [1]. Just 7 days later, the Environmental Protection Agency (EPA) declared that the air and water were safe; however, the exact nature of what was in this enormous amount of dust was not fully understood [2]. Long-term results from exposed rescue workers, locals, and those involved in the cleanup suggest that the EPA's decision was both premature and inappropriate. Over the subsequent 12 to 18 months, significant amounts of dust were deposited across Brooklyn, exposing additional millions [3]. In addition to the initial dust exposure from the collapse of the towers, fires—which reached over 1000 °C—in dust-covered rubble created a vast array of chemicals not originally in the dust and spread them throughout the area for several months prior to being fully extinguished in December 2001 [4]. Despite millions of homes in the area, there was little effort to contain and immediately clean up the area, as it was not declared a toxic waste site [1]. In fact, after the EPA decided to regulate ground zero and the cleanup, the New York City Department of Health simply suggested using a wet mop to clean the area [1].

Without a legal requirement to remove dust, many people received significant indoor exposures every day for months [1]. This was further exacerbated by the fact that the dust was 10–1000 times more easily aerosolized than normal dusts, allowing easy re-suspension and recontamination [3]. This was likely a result of being smaller, with more than 50% of particles <53 μm in diameter, a size pattern unique to WTC [3]. This dust migrated indoors and was further compounded by the fact that these characteristics made it more easily inhalable therefore magnifying its

M. Kostrubiak
University of Vermont College of Medicine, Burlington, VT, USA
e-mail: marc.kostrubiak@stonybrook.edu

impacts and allowing particles to reach smaller airways [3, 5]. In addition to straight inhalation, dust was subject to both dietary and non-dietary ingestion due to deposition and suspension in homes and workplaces [6].

Despite the initial EPA safety claim, we now know that understanding the composition of the dust and the various kinds of exposure is critical for efforts to understand the significant health effects and determine research avenues for future treatments. Presently, we know that locals and first responders have high incidences of aerodigestive issues including gastroesophageal reflux onset or exacerbation, interstitial lung diseases, sinusitis, and various asthma-like illnesses [1]. Higher rates of solid tumors and hematological cancers have also been found in this group [1, 7]). Finally, it is clear that mental health issues arose and remain in many who were affected directly or indirectly [1, 7, 8, 9]. While this is only a brief summary of the range of effects, it is clear that the 9/11 attacks have affected the health of thousands for nearly two decades and will probably continue to do so for the rest of their lives. Furthermore, understanding the exact nature of the dust and related disease states may help treat thousands around the world with various industrial, military, and environmental exposures.

On September 16 and 17, three initial samples of dust were taken from wind-protected areas and provide much of our understanding of the dust composition [6]. The majority of the highly alkaline (pH 9–11.5) dust consisted of pulverized building materials: concrete, gypsum, synthetic vitreous fibers, various metals, and asbestos [6]. Overall composition structure can be broken down to between 37 and 50% non-fiber content, 40% glass fibers, between 9.2 and 20% cellulose, and 0.8 to 3% chrysolite asbestos [6]. Combustion created radionuclides, ionic species, polycyclic aromatic hydrocarbons, and polychlorinated biphenyls (PCBs), among other organic byproducts that became significant components of dust [1, 4, 6]. The particles were mostly (52.21–63.60%) greater than 53 μm in diameter with between 0.8 and 1.30% less than 2.5 μm [6]. The smallest components of the dust, with diameters less than 2.5 pm (known as $PM_{2.5}$), are particularly important as they play a stronger role in cardiovascular disease processes than do larger particles [5, 10].

Geographic and Temporal Aspects

The declared New York City disaster area included all of Manhattan, south of Houston Street, and all areas within 1.5 miles of the location where the World Trade Center once stood. This includes a minimal portion of Governor's Island and the DUMBO neighborhood and parts of Brooklyn Heights and Vinegar Hill in Brooklyn. People who lived in this area for at least 4 days in the 4 months, or 30 days prior to July 31, 2002, are eligible for the World Trade Center Health Program; however, as previously mentioned, the dust spread was not limited to a 1.5 mile radius [11]. In the first 12–18 h, the dust and smoke cloud largely dispersed toward the east and subsequently southeast across Brooklyn [6]. On that first day, the plume dispersion was modeled as traveling much further south than the disaster area—possibly as far as through Brighton Beach and on onto Rockaway Point [4, 11]. The plume modeling output covers about half of Brooklyn. Unfortunately, the spread of dust was subsequently enlarged on September 13 when the south/southeast winds gave way to an east/northeasterly flow exposing parts of Manhattan up to East Harlem, Roosevelt Island, southern parts of the Bronx, and much of Queens [11].

Luckily, despite this large area, the exposures outside of lower Manhattan are presently not thought to have been significant but are to be noted as long-term health effects may still arise [4]. Furthermore, while the winds may have changed on the 13th and increased the potential exposure area, the most intense exposures were only during the first 12 h, and burning jet fuel and building fires were put out within 1.5–2 days (although as previous mentioned, various debris fires last until December) [4]. Exposures have been classified based on severity with category 1 accounting for the first 12 h, category 2 then lasts until 2 days afterward, category 3 for days 3 to 13, and category 4 for days 14 through December 29, 2001 [4]. While some aspects of exposure in these categories—such as gaseous inhalation—remain unknown, only categories 1 and 2 were exposed to jet fuel and building fires. Due to rain on day 4—September 15—dust re-suspension was generally caused by cleanup efforts and, in particular, moving trucks and large equipment rather than winds which had been able to stir up loose dry dust beforehand [4]. This fortunate change made category 4 exposures smaller and much more localized [4]. While many locals were afflicted in the first 12 h—category 1—large numbers left the area and did not return to their homes or work for a week, thus escaping the time period for category 2 exposure [1]. Therefore many of the locals may have avoided the two most serious outdoor exposure categories. After the second rainfall on day 14—September 25— re-suspension was uncommon and resulted in very limited exposures [4]. Due to the inconsistent nature of indoor cleanup, it has been assigned its own category—5— without a known or consistent end point.

Due to the unprecedented nature of the September 11 attacks, testing for pollutants, particularly near ground zero, was not immediately performed and thus early levels (categories 1–3) of various chemicals remain uncertain: asbestos was not assessed until the 14th; benzene, PCBs, lead, dioxins, and volatile organic compounds (VOCs) on the 16th, $PM_{2.5}$ (particulate matter smaller than or equal to 2.5 microns in diameter) on the 21st, and PAHs on the 23rd [5, 12, 13].

Nonorganics, Metals, Ions, and Asbestos

Building materials found include vermiculite, paint, plaster, foam, lead, calcite, wood, glass, and asbestos [6]. Glass found varied in size from 1 μm to over 10 μm in width and ranged in length from 5 to 100 μm. It was often coated with other materials, bringing in other components, frequently calcium, silicon, and sulfur, when inhaled or consumed [6]. These elements are associated with pulmonary toxicity and various potentially fatal pulmonary disease states such as silicosis, which can reduce gas exchange and potentially decrease surface tension within alveoli [14, 15].

Dust samples taken on September 16 and 17 contained a variety of ions in varying concentrations. Sulfate (SO_4^{2-}) (Fig. 1), most likely from fires, and calcium were present in the greatest amounts by weight although a variety of other biologically active ions were isolated (Table 1).

Health considerations of exposure to these ions vary from insignificant to potentially severe. Long-term fluoride exposure can cause skeletal fluorosis, while short-term effects include bronchiolar ulceration and other lung injury [16]. Fluoride is also reactive and could have become a number of highly toxic substances such as oxygen difluoride in the immediate aftermath [16]. Many of these ions, including the most common by mass—sulfate—can create highly oxidizing species and free radicals, creating oxidative stress [17]. Sulfates were particularly common in the $PM_{2.5}$ portion and may thus have a stronger cardiovascular impact than otherwise expected [5, 10]. Nitrates, the other polyatomic ion (NO_3^-), can cause hypotension and headaches and have been found to be potentially beneficial in some cases but may increase risk of stroke and heart disease-related mortality due to chronic exposure, as well as being considered "probably carcinogenic to humans" [18]. While most people were not chronically exposed to dust, all of these long-term effects may still impact local residents via category 5 exposure or the more severe, albeit briefer categories 1–4 exposures.

Fig. 1 Structure of a sulfate ion

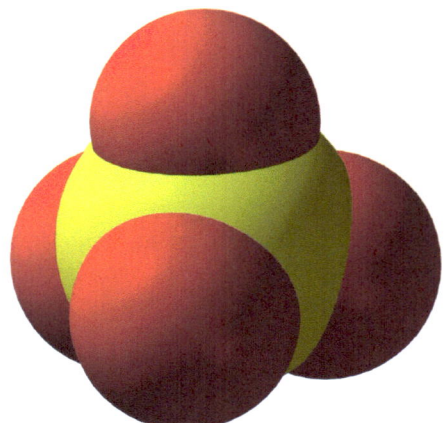

Table 1 Ion concentrations in the dust as found by [6]

Ion	Minimum (ng/g)	Maximum (ng/g)
Fluoride	Not detectable	220
Chloride	220	800
Nitrate	Not detectable	330
Sulfate	35,200	42,100
Calcium	14,000	18,200
Sodium	130	400
Potassium	60	270

Asbestos is widely recognized as a potent carcinogen and a factor in the vast majority of mesothelioma cases (National Cancer Institute) as well as recently recognized contributions to laryngeal, ovarian, and many other cancers [19]. Even short-term limited exposure, as short as a 16 h, has been associated with mesothelioma later in life and is thus a huge concern for first responders and the local population [20]. Outdoor dusts varied from 0.8 to 3% asbestos, whereas indoor samples were all less than 1%. The outdoor dusts may raise concerns, and while the indoor samples had low asbestos concentrations, they may have provided much longer exposure durations [3, 6]. A risk assessment based on outdoor exposures for a month found an increased cancer risk of only 1/40th of the lifetime risk and thus negligible; however, as established, both outdoor and indoor exposures may have lasted significantly longer [12, 13]. Furthermore, this assessment is limited by using data from several days after 9/11 and may be using artificially low asbestos levels, and thus others recommend long-term monitoring and follow-up studies [21].

Overall elemental analysis showed levels consistent with the source of the dust and included relatively high levels of titanium (Table 2) and lead from paints, but

Table 2 The minimum and maximum levels of metals highlight some important health considerations

Element	Minimum (ng/g)	Maximum (ng/g)
Lithium	22,650	29,520
Beryllium	2638	3754
Magnesium	110,300	179,000
Aluminum	558,800	908,700
Titanium	1,485,000	1,797,000
Vanadium	33,890	42,610
Chromium	142,600	182,000
Manganese	565,100	828,100
Cobalt	7230	10,460
Nickel	41,140	47,290
Copper	133,500	336,300
Zinc	1,718,000	2,992,000
Gallium	26,990	34,060
Arsenic	2464	2792
Rubidium	18,630	21,710
Strontium	478,900	720,800
Silver	1945	2565
Cadmium	5695	8454
Cesium	1085	1327
Barium	365,300	406,500
Thallium	905	1954
Lead	142,400	483,500
Bismuth	1087	1466
Uranium	3920	4213

undetectably low levels of mercury [6]. The most common element, zinc, has unclear effects. It has been found to be minimally toxic in one study [22], while being implicated in antioxidation, DNA damage, and membrane stability deficits [23]. In terms of quantity and deposition, some elements were very consistent, whereas others had large variation; thus, exposures to certain elements may have varied greatly depending on temporal and locational effects.

Titanium, the second most common element in the samples (by ng/g), when inhaled, particularly in conjunction with iron, is suspected to be a key component of Iraq-Afghanistan War Lung Injury [24]. It has also been linked to interstitial pneumonitis, peribronchial inflammation, and pulmonary fibrosis [25].

While lead was high in dust samples, it was similar to levels in cities suffering from old leaded fuel combustion [26]. However, in the immediate aftermath of the attacks and subsequent collapse of the towers, persons were exposed to high levels of lead, but it faded quickly over several days and was quickly dissipated over several blocks from ground zero. Long-term health effects are believed to be limited to children of women who were pregnant in the immediate vicinity [11].

Chromium levels were elevated up to four times greater than background however remained under OSHA health guidelines [11]. Chromium VI is a carcinogen associated with lung and nasal cancers; however, Cr III is an essential nutrient and dietary supplement [11, 27]. The body is able to reduce chromium VI to III, and it is unlikely to have had long-term impacts at these low levels [27].

Additionally, arsenic and cadmium were relatively low but still at potentially concerning levels [6]. Arsenic, a highly toxic metal, has been linked to a wide variety of health concerns including neurological and cognitive dysfunction, diabetes, hypertension-related cardiovascular disease and strokes, cancers, and chronic respiratory disease [28–30]. With such a broad and severe set of symptoms, it is of long-term significance for a large portion of the exposed population. Cadmium generates oxidative stress and is thus an International Agency for Research on Cancer (IARC) class 1 carcinogen and able to cause renal failure via tubular proteinuria ([31, 32]; EPA). Furthermore cadmium inhalation has been associated with COPD, chronic obstructive lung disease, emphysema, rhinitis and even lung cancers [33].

Aluminum, another major constituent, was once thought to be protective against silicosis [34]. Unfortunately, it lacks the previously theorized protective benefits and can instead contribute to cardiovascular diseases and Alzheimer's disease [34].

Similarly, manganese found in the dust can be deposited in the brain after inhalation and accumulated preferentially parts of the brain including the striatum and pineal gland [35]. By accumulating in these areas, it appears to modulate dopamine systems and can therefore impact behavior, including motor defects, along with its general neurotoxic effects [35]. Furthermore, only 3 weeks of inhalation, a short time for ground zero locals, was shown to cause lung injury and change dopamine receptor expression in rats [35].

Organics: PAHs, Pesticides, VOCs, and Dioxins

Analysis of outdoor dust provides an interesting picture of organic materials found in WTC dust, both from initial dispersal and from the subsequent months of fires in ground zero rubble. The high cellulose content, about 20% of the dust, is attributed to paper and office materials that were distributed by the explosions and collapse of the towers [6]. The only pesticides in the test that were detected were hexachlorobenzene (HCB) (Fig. 2) and 4,4-dichlorodiphenyldichloroethylene (DDE) and mirex (Table 3) [6]. While there was high relative variability, overall the compositions are quite similar.

Hexachlorobenzene (HCB) is categorized as a possible human carcinogen, is globally banned, and has been illegal in the USA since 1966 but was still found in the WTC dust. HCB has been found to cause liver and breast cancer in rats [36]. It has also believed to cause hypothyroidism with even subchronic exposures [37], oxidative stress, and DNA damage [38].

Fig. 2 The relatively simple organic structure of HCB

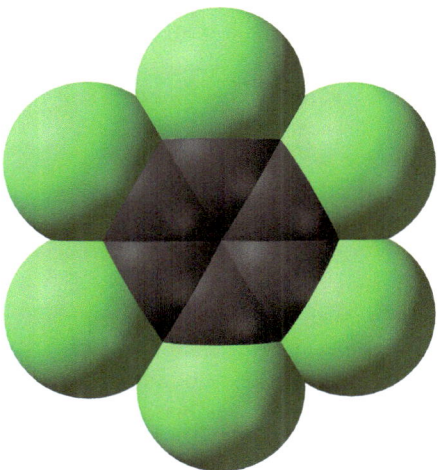

Table 3 Fortunately most concerning pesticides were not found, although the presence of HCB, DDE, and mirex remain significant

Pesticide	Minimum (ng/g)	Maximum (ng/g)
Hexachlorobenzene	0.9	1.9
Heptachlor	Not detected	Not detected
4,4-DDE	1.3	3.0
2,4-DDT	Not detected	Not detected
4,4-DDT	Not detected	Not detected
Mirex	Not detected	0.8
Total chlordane pesticides	3.1	5.6

Like HCB, mirex has been illegal for decades with its last allowed use in the USA occurring in 1978, 2 years after sale was outlawed. Animal models have similarly shown a significant carcinogenic potential for mirex. Prenatal exposure to mirex is believed to impair neural development and cause cognitive deficits in children [39] along with general neurotoxic effects.

4,4-DDE, a breakdown product of dichlorodiphenyltrichloroethane (DDT) (Fig. 3), is highly lipophilic, bioaccumulates readily, and is neurotoxic [40, 41]. The only major source of excretion is actually through breastmilk—thus potentially affecting those who were not even alive on 9/11 [40]. Prenatal and pediatric exposure has been associated with visual processing defects and general neuronal apoptosis [41, 42]. Like HCB, it is another IARC class 2 carcinogen—possibly causing cancer in humans. Further, DDE is an endocrine disruptor that can hinder spermatogenesis, potentially causing type 1 diabetes and hepatic lipid dysfunction [43, 44].

Polycyclic aromatic hydrocarbon (PAH) levels varied heavily from sample to sample; however, the profile of various PAHs was consistent, implying a common source but unequal dispersion of gross PAHs over the region [6, 45]. PAH exposure is quite concerning as they have been linked to a variety of cancers including lung, skin, kidney, and bladder among others [46]. With their aromatic carbon rings, PAHs and their metabolites are able to bind directly to DNA causing mutations [47]. PAH-induced mutations are believed to be heritable and can actually be passed to children via breastmilk [47].

Overall, polycyclic aromatic hydrocarbons (PAHs) (Fig. 4) accounted for more than 0.1% of the dust mass (Table 4)—a high level that has both short- and long-term health implications [6]. Generally, relative levels of PAHs in dust were elevated close to ground zero and particularly near fires [6]. Levels of PAHs, along with polychlorinated biphenyls (PCBs), polychlorinated naphthalenes (PCNs), and polybrominated diphenyl ethers (PDBEs) were markedly higher within 1 km of ground zero and declined to background levels by 3.5 km (2.2 miles) [48]. This radius does extend past the official WTC disaster area. While

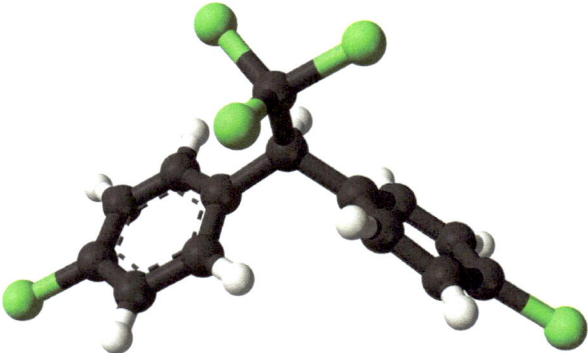

Fig. 3 DDT and its breakdown product DDE are of particular concern for those exposed to WTC dust

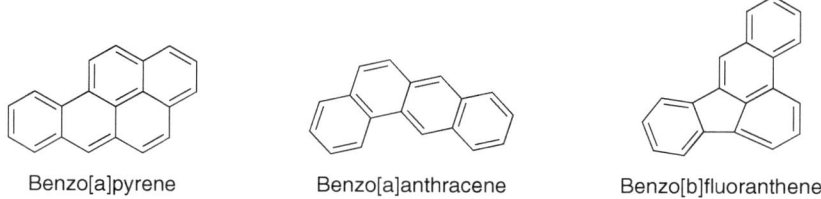

Benzo[a]pyrene   Benzo[a]anthracene   Benzo[b]fluoranthene

Fig. 4 PAHs like the ones shown tend to have similar structures and pose similar threats including potential DNA damage

Table 4 Significant levels of several different PAHs were found albeit with significant variability from sample to sample

Compound (PAHs)	Minimum (ng/g)	Maximum (ng/g)
Fluorene	2620	32,200
Phenanthrene	22,300	44,100
Fluoranthene	13,700	40,300
Benzo(a)pyrene	12,100	23,000
Benzo(b+k)fluoranthene	15,600	36,600
Total PAH's	218,100	383,300

PAHs are not acutely toxic, chronic exposure has been reported to cause chronic bronchitis, coughs, and dermatitis and thus add to the litany of pulmonary threats found in the WTC dusts [47].

Over 90,000 L of jet fuel and subsequent fires contributed to creating a vast array of volatile and semi-volatile organic compounds (VOCs and SVOCs) [6]. Many VOCs are also categorized as PAHs and share many of the same characteristics and accordingly health concerns. Lioy et al. [6] tested for 300 of these hydrocarbons and found significant amounts of many of them. Especially concerning was the presence of phthalate esters, which accounted for over 100 µg/g in the samples. This particular group of organics has been found to cause birth defects, potentially through their endocrine-disrupting impacts [49]. This antiandrogen action has been further associated with testicular and breast cancers [50, 51]. Phthalate exposure has also been correlated with obesity, a particularly troubling impact as many affected by 9/11 suffer from lung function declines and may therefore have a reduced ability to exercise [52].

Other significant VOCs include naphthalene: 5.3–7.5 µg/g and fluorene: up to 50,000 µg/g, both of which are also PAHs [6]. Naphthalenes in general are another potential human carcinogen (IARC class 3) and have been found to cause respiratory lesions and tumors in animal studies [53]. Methylnaphthalene has been found to cause pulmonary alveolar proteinosis [54]. Despite these concerns, it is difficult to assess whether naphthalene exposures are significant as it is nearly ubiquitous due to a variety of applications such as mothballs, deodorants, and other household products. Therefore, WTC-related exposures might be marginal compared to life-long exposures [53].

Many of the VOCs found were paraffins and cycloparaffins from the JP-8 jet fuel and subsequent combustion [6]. Long-term paraffin exposure may be associated with chronic lipoid pneumonia [55]. Overall, it is difficult to assess dangers from VOCs, as many have not undergone significant research. However, current research has found associations between VOCs and various cancers, neurological effects, liver and kidney damage and asthma and allergies [56, 57, 58].

An analysis of indoor dust found that PCB levels were comparable to outdoor levels, and even similar to an unaffected area [45]. While PCBs have been illegal for decades, since the World Trade Center was built in the 1970s, it likely housed various electronic components that became a source of PCBs [11]. The collapse of the towers destroyed two electrical substations located underground that contained about 490,000 L of PCB containing oil [48]. PCBs are another class B2 probable human carcinogen, particularly affecting the liver [11]. Overall, levels in the air after 9/11 remained below limits set by NIOSH [11]. Unfortunately, hexachlorobenzene (and heptachlor, which was undetected in outdoor dusts) levels were elevated in these same indoor dust samples [45]. Conversely, several aforementioned organochloride pesticides—4,4-DDT, 2,4-DDT, 4,4-DDE, and mirex—were actually well below ambient levels [45]. Finally, just like in outdoor dusts, PAH levels varied heavily but remained relatively constant in proportion to one another [45].

Polychlorinated dibenzodioxins (PCDDs) (Figs. 5 and 6), known simply as dioxins, were another unfortunate component of the dust, although levels may not have been significantly higher than background [6]. However it is still important to consider their effects due to their long half-lives and being considered class 1 carcinogens by the IARC. PCDD exposure may cause hypertension, atherosclerosis, thyroid function, diabetes, and central and peripheral neurological impairment and birth defects in children [59–61]. These various impacts are often only associated with dioxins in cases where patients experienced high exposure due to the

Fig. 5 PCDDs are of particular concern due to their strong carcinogenic qualities

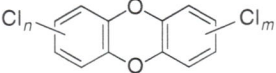

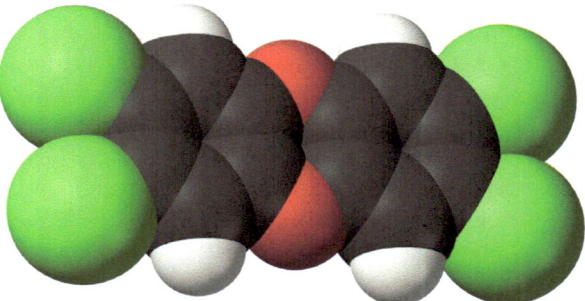

Fig. 6 PCDD structure shares commonalities with the other concerning organics such as PAHs and HCB but has unique characteristics such as their central oxygen atoms (*red*)

time delay and the symptoms nonspecific multifactorial nature; thus they may be under-reported [61]. As dioxins have severe long-term consequences, the possibility that exposures were elevated from dust in the air and indoors suggests the need for long-term monitoring.

Conclusion

The World Trade Center disaster on September 11, 2001, created a unique environmental hazard exposing many to a complex amalgam of chemicals through inhalation of dust for months. Many of the components in the dust are carcinogens and have a variety of cardiopulmonary impacts. In fact, 6 months afterward, 38% of fire and rescue workers reported a severe cough from their exposure [4]. Furthermore, many of the chemicals are acutely toxic as well as causing long-term damage to important organs such as the liver and kidneys. While we still do not know the effects of hundreds of elements and organic chemicals in the dust, it is important to follow those exposed to WTC dust and be aware of the various disease end points possible. Further, following those affected may prove beneficial for our understanding of many poorly researched chemicals as well as helping treatment for other exposures such as burn pits in Iraq or industrial sites especially prominent in South East Asia.

References

1. Reibman J, Levy-carrick N, Miles T, et al. Destruction of the world trade center towers. lessons learned from an environmental health disaster. Ann Am Thorac Soc. 2016;13(5):577–83.
2. Environmental Protection Agency. Environmental news. whitman details ongoing agency efforts to monitor disaster sites, Contribute to Cleanup effort. Newsroom. EPA, 18 Sept 2001. Web.
3. Yiin L-M, Millette JR, Vette A, Ilacqua V, Quan C, Gorczynski J, Kendall M, Chen LC, Weisel CP, Buckley B, Yang I, Lioy PJ. Comparisons of the dust/smoke particulate that settled inside the surrounding buildings and outside on the streets of southern New York City after the collapse of the World Trade Center, September 11, 2001. J Air Waste Manage Assoc. 2004;54(5):515–28.
4. Lioy PJ, Pellizzari E, Prezant D. The World Trade Center aftermath and its effects on health: understanding and learning through human-exposure science. Environ Sci Technol. 2006;40(22):6876–85.
5. Olson DA, Norris GA, Landis MS, Vette AF. Chemical characterization of ambient particulate matter near the World Trade Center: elemental carbon, organic carbon, and mass reconstruction. Environ Sci Technol. 2004;38(17):4465–73.
6. Lioy PJ, Weisel CP, Millette JR, et al. Characterization of the dust/smoke aerosol that settled east of the World Trade Center (WTC) in lower Manhattan after the collapse of the WTC 11 September 2001. Environ Health Perspect. 2002;110(7):703–14.
7. Centers for Disease Control and Prevention. WTC health program at a glance. 2015. Available from http://www.cdc.gov/wtc/ataglance/html. Accessed 20 June 2016.
8. Farfel M, Digrande L, Brackbill R, et al. An overview of 9/11 experiences and respiratory and mental health conditions among World Trade Center Health Registry enrollees. J Urban Health. 2008;85(6):880–909.

9. Hoven CW, Duarte CS, Lucas CP, et al. Psychopathology among New York city public school children 6 months after September 11. Arch Gen Psychiatry. 2005;62(5):545–52.
10. Mcgee JK, Chen LC, Cohen MD, et al. Chemical analysis of World Trade Center fine particulate matter for use in toxicologic assessment. Environ Health Perspect. 2003;111(7):972–80.
11. United States. Environmental Protection Agency. National Center for Environmental Assessment Office of Research and Development. Exposure and Human Health Evaluation of Airborne Pollution from the World Trade Center Disaster. N.p.: n.p.;2002.
12. Lorber M, Gibb H, Grant L, Pinto J, Pleil J, Cleverly D. Assessment of inhalation exposures and potential health risks to the general population that resulted from the collapse of the World Trade Center towers. Risk Anal. 2007a;27(5):1203–21.
13. Lorber M, Gibb H, Grant LD, Pinto JP, Pleil J, Cleverly D. Assessment of inhalation exposures and potential health risks to the general population that resulted from the collapse of the world trade center towers. Risk Anal. 2007b;27(5):1203–21.
14. Drummond G, Bevan R, Harrison P. A comparison of the results from intra-pleural and intra-peritoneal studies with those from inhalation and intratracheal tests for the assessment of pulmonary responses to inhalable dusts and fibres. Regul Toxicol Pharmacol. 2016;81:89–105.
15. Bhattacharjee P, Paul S, Bhattacharjee P. Risk of occupational exposure to asbestos, silicon and arsenic on pulmonary disorders: Understanding the genetic-epigenetic interplay and future prospects. Environ Res. 2016;147:425–34.
16. F Fluorides, Hydrogen Fluoride and Fluorine. Environmental health and medicine education. Agency for toxic substances and disease registry, n.d. Web.
17. Pham-huy LA, He H, Pham-huy C. Free radicals, antioxidants in disease and health. Int J Biomed Sci. 2008;4(2):89–96.
18. Nitrate/Nitrite Toxicity. Environmental health and medicine education. Agency for Toxic Substances and Disease Registry, 05 Dec 2015. Web.
19. Scherpereel A. Asbestos and respiratory diseases. Presse Med. 2016;45(1):117–32.
20. Leigh J, Driscoll T. Malignant mesothelioma in Australia, 1945–2002. Int J Occup Environ Health. 2003;9(3):206–17.
21. Landrigan PJ, Lioy PJ, Thurston G, Gertrud B, Chen LC, Chillrud SN, Gavett SH, Georgopoulos PG, Geyh AS, Levin S, Perera F, Rappaport SM, Small C. Health and Environmental Consequences of the World Trade Center Disaster. Environ Health Perspect. 2004;112(6):731–9.
22. Morimoto Y, Izumi H, Yoshiura Y, et al. Evaluation of pulmonary toxicity of zinc oxide nanoparticles following inhalation and intratracheal instillation. Int J Mol Sci. 2016;17(8):1241.
23. Lee SH, Wang TY, Hong JH, Cheng TJ, Lin CY. NMR-based metabolomics to determine acute inhalation effects of nano- and fine-sized ZnO particles in the rat lung. Nanotoxicology. 2016;10(7):924–34.
24. Szema AM, Schmidt MP, Lanzirotti A, Harrington AD, Lyubsky S, Reeder RJ, Schoonen MA. Titanium and iron in lung of a soldier with nonspecific interstitial pneumonitis and bronchiolitis after returning from Iraq. J Occup Environ Med. 2012;54(1):1–2.
25. Szema AM, Reeder RJ, Harrington AD, Schmidt M, Liu J, Golightly M, Rueb T, Hamidi SA. Iraq dust is respirable, sharp, and metal-laden and induces lung inflammation with fibrosis in mice via IL-2 upregulation and depletion of regulatory T Cells. J Occup Environ Med. 2014;56(3):243–51.
26. Lioy PJ, Yiin LM, Adgate J, Weisel C, Rhoads GG. The effectiveness of a home cleaning intervention strategy in reducing potential dust and lead exposures. J Expo Anal Environ Epidemiol. 1998;8(1):17–35.
27. Rowbotham AL, Levy LS. Chromium in the environment: an evaluation of exposure of the UK general population and possible adverse health effects. J Toxicol Environ Health B Crit Rev. 2000;3(3):145–78.
28. Chiou HY, Huang WI, Su CL, Chang SF, Hsu YH, Chen CJ. Dose-response relationship between prevalence of cerebrovascular disease and ingested inorganic arsenic. Stroke. 1997;28(9):1717–23.

29. Hendryx M. Mortality from heart, respiratory, and kidney disease in coal mining areas of Appalachia. Int Arch Occup Environ Health. 2009;82(2):243–9.
30. Tseng CH, Chong CK, Tseng CP, et al. Long-term arsenic exposure and ischemic heart disease in arseniasis-hyperendemic villages in Taiwan. Toxicol Lett. 2003;137(1-2):15–21.
31. Maret W, Moulis JM. The bioinorganic chemistry of cadmium in the context of its toxicity. Met Ions Life Sci. 2013;11:1–29.
32. Safety and Health Topics Cadmium. Case studies in environmental medicine. United States Department of Labor Occupational Safety and Health Administration, n.d. Web.
33. Cadmium Toxicity. Environmental health and medicine education. Agency for Toxic Substances & Disease Registry, 05 Dec 2015. Web.
34. Peters S, Reid A, Fritschi L, De klerk N, Musk AW. Long-term effects of aluminium dust inhalation. Occup Environ Med. 2013;70(12):864–8.
35. Saputra D, Chang J, Lee BJ, Yoon JH, Kim J, Lee K. Short-term manganese inhalation decreases brain dopamine transporter levels without disrupting motor skills in rats. J Toxicol Sci. 2016;41(3):391–402.
36. Delisle A, Ferraris E, Plante I. Chronic exposure to hexachlorobenzene results in down-regulation of connexin43 in the breast. Environ Res. 2015;143(Pt A):229–40.
37. Chalouati H, Gamet-payrastre L, Saad MB. Irreversible thyroid disruption induced after sub-chronic exposure to hexachlorobenzene in male rats. Toxicol Ind Health. 2016;32(5):822–31.
38. Chalouati H, Boutet E, Metais B, Fouche E, Ben sâad MM, Gamet-payrastre L. DNA damage and oxidative stress induced at low doses by the fungicide hexachlorobenzene in human intestinal Caco-2 cells. Toxicol Mech Methods. 2015;25(6):448–58.
39. Puertas R, Lopez-espinosa MJ, Cruz F, et al. Prenatal exposure to mirex impairs neurodevelopment at age of 4 years. Neurotoxicology. 2010;31(1):154–60.
40. Waliszewski SM, Melo-santiesteban G, Villalobos-pietrini R, et al. Breast milk excretion Kinetic of b-HCH, pp'DDE and pp'DDT. Bull Environ Contam Toxicol. 2009;83(6):869–73.
41. Wnuk A, Rzemieniec J, Litwa E, Lasoń W, Krzeptowski W, Wójtowicz AK, Kajta M. The crucial involvement of Retinoid X receptors in DDE neurotoxicity. Neurotox Res. 2016;29(1):155–72.
42. Cartier C, Muckle G, Jacobson SW, et al. Prenatal and 5-year p,p'-DDE exposures are associated with altered sensory processing in school-aged children in Nunavik: a visual evoked potential study. Neurotoxicology. 2014;44:8–16.
43. Quan C, Shi Y, Wang C, Wang C, Yang K. p,p'-DDE damages spermatogenesis via phospholipid hydroperoxide glutathione peroxidase depletion and mitochondria apoptosis pathway. Environ Toxicol. 2016;31(5):593–600.
44. Rodríguez-Alcalá LM, Sá C, Pimentel LL, Pestana D, Teixeira D, Faria A, Calhau C, Gomes A. Endocrine disruptor DDE Associated with a high-fat diet enhances the impairment of liver fatty acid composition in rats. J Agric Food Chem. 2015;63(42):9341–8.
45. Offenberg JH, Eisenreich SJ, Gigliotti CL, et al. Persistent organic pollutants in dusts that settled indoors in lower Manhattan after September 11, 2001. J Expo Anal Environ Epidemiol. 2004;14(2):164–72.
46. Boström CE, Gerde P, Hanberg A, et al. Cancer risk assessment, indicators, and guidelines for polycyclic aromatic hydrocarbons in the ambient air. Environ Health Perspect. 2002;110(Suppl 3):451–88.
47. Toxicity of Polycyclic Aromatic Hydrocarbons. Case studies in environmental medicine. Agency for Toxic Substances and Disease Registry, 01 July 2009. Web.
48. Butt CM, Diamond ML, Truong J, Ikonomou MG, Helm PA, Stern GA. Semivolatile organic compounds in window films from lower Manhattan after the September 11th World Trade Center attacks. Environ Sci Technol. 2004;38(13):3514–24.
49. Albert O, Jégou B. A critical assessment of the endocrine susceptibility of the human testis to phthalates from fetal life to adulthood. Hum Reprod Update. 2014;20(2):231–49.
50. López-carrillo L, Hernández-ramírez RU, Calafat AM, et al. Exposure to phthalates and breast cancer risk in northern Mexico. Environ Health Perspect. 2010;118(4):539–44.

51. National Research Council (US) Committee on the Health Risks of Phthalates. Phthalates and cumulative risk assessment, the task ahead. Washington, DC: National Academies Press; 2008.
52. Hou JW, Lin CL, Tsai YA, et al. The effects of phthalate and nonylphenol exposure on body size and secondary sexual characteristics during puberty. Int J Hyg Environ Health. 2015;218(7):603–15.
53. Batterman S, Chin JY, Jia C, et al. Sources, concentrations, and risks of naphthalene in indoor and outdoor air. Indoor Air. 2012;22(4):266–78.
54. Murata Y, Emi Y, Denda A, Konishi Y. Ultrastructural analysis of pulmonary alveolar proteinosis induced by methylnaphthalene in mice. Exp Toxicol Pathol. 1992;44(1):47–54.
55. Han C, Liu L, Du S, et al. Investigation of rare chronic lipoid pneumonia associated with occupational exposure to paraffin aerosol. J Occup Health. 2016;58(5):482–8.
56. Tagiyeva N, Sheikh A. Domestic exposure to volatile organic compounds in relation to asthma and allergy in children and adults. Expert Rev Clin Immunol. 2014;10(12):1611–39.
57. Loh MM, Levy JI, Spengler JD, Houseman EA, Bennett DH. Ranking cancer risks of organic hazardous air pollutants in the United States. Environ Health Perspect. 2007;115(8):1160–8.
58. Nurmatov UB, Tagiyeva N, Semple S, Devereux G, Sheikh A. Volatile organic compounds and risk of asthma and allergy: a systematic review. Eur Respir Rev. 2015;24(135):92–101.
59. Arisawa K, Takeda H, Mikasa H. Background exposure to PCDDs/PCDFs/PCBs and its potential health effects: a review of epidemiologic studies. J Med Investig. 2005;52(1-2):10–21.
60. Pavuk M, Schecter AJ, Akhtar FZ, Michalek JE. Serum 2,3,7,8-tetrachlorodibenzo-p-dioxin (TCDD) levels and thyroid function in Air Force veterans of the Vietnam War. Ann Epidemiol. 2003;13(5):335–43.
61. Pelclová D, Urban P, Preiss J, et al. Adverse health effects in humans exposed to 2,3,7,8-tetrachlorodibenzo-p-dioxin (TCDD). Rev Environ Health. 2006;21(2):119–38.

The Mental Health of Children and Adolescents Exposed to 9/11: Lessons Learned and Still to be Learned

Talya Greene, Raz Gross, Lawrence Amsel, and Christina W. Hoven

Introduction

The events of September 11, 2001 had, and will continue to have, a profound economic, political, and psychological impact on the entire population of the United States. However, those exposed to the events of 9/11 as children or adolescents had a very distinct experience, with unique sequelae. As Klassen et al. [1] noted in a related context, 'Children are not just small adults'. Thousands of children and adolescents had direct experience of the attack on the World Trade Center (WTC), and

T. Greene (✉)
Department of Community Mental Health, University of Haifa,
199 Aba Khoushy Avenue, Haifa 3498838, Israel
e-mail: tgreene@univ.haifa.ac.il

R. Gross
Division of Psychiatry, The Chaim Sheba Medical Center, Tel Hashomer, Israel

Department of Epidemiology and Preventive Medicine, Sackler Faculty of Medicine,
Tel Aviv University, PO Box 39040, Tel Aviv 6997801, Israel
e-mail: razg@post.tau.ac.il

L. Amsel
Clinical Psychiatry, College of Physicians and Surgeons, Columbia University,
New York, NY 10027, USA

New York State Psychiatric Institute, New York, NY 10032, USA

New York Presbyterian Hospital, New York, NY 10032, USA
e-mail: lamsel01@gmail.com

C.W. Hoven
Epidemiology and Psychiatry, Columbia University-NYSPI, New York, NY 10032, USA

Department of Child Psychiatric Epidemiology, Columbia University-NYSPI,
New York, NY 10032, USA
e-mail: HOVEN@nyspi.columbia.edu

© Springer International Publishing AG 2018
A.M. Szema (ed.), *World Trade Center Pulmonary Diseases and Multi-Organ System Manifestations*, DOI 10.1007/978-3-319-59372-2_9

many others knew someone who was injured, killed, or directly exposed. But even those young people who lived far from New York City on 9/11 were impacted by this unprecedented disaster and continue to experience its ripple effects on their mental and physical well-being to this day [2].

A systematic review looking back over a decade of research concerning children living in the vicinity of the WTC found that they were indeed uniquely affected by this untoward event [3]. Yet, it is important to recognize that while the WTC attack generated a significant body of literature focused on its mental health impact on adults, there has been a much less thorough research approach to those exposed as children and adolescents [4, 5]. Moreover, this limitation is being perpetuated today in the disproportionately small amount of funds allocated to services and research targeting those under 18 years of age on September 11, 2001, through the Zadroga Act, a congressionally mandated mechanism created to provide services to, and an understanding of, physical and mental health-related outcomes among those exposed.

In 2019, the youngest of those exposed will reach adulthood, carrying that experience with them. It seems useful, therefore, to look back at studies that did investigate the mental health effects of 9/11 on those exposed as children or adolescents, in order to understand what was done, what might have been done differently, and what yet remains to be done. Our intention here is to provide a critical overview of the studies that investigated psychopathological outcomes attributed to the WTC attack among youth ages 0–18 years on 9/11, as well as to identify what else might have been done and what still needs to be done to fill the knowledge gaps. Because, to date, very little has been done to address the physical health-related consequences in youth, the methodologies of studies included here focus on those directly or indirectly exposed and their measured outcomes, ranging from isolated psychiatric symptoms to full psychiatric disorders and from documenting patterns of substance use to prevalence of substance use disorders (SUD). Importantly, the intentions of the investigators of those studies were always to identify which categories of youth were most affected, how they were affected, and which risk factors contributed to the outcomes. We present this overview for the purpose of asking the readers and ourselves what lessons have been learned and how might the scientific research community better serve public health in the future?

Children Are Not Just Small Adults

Obviously, children and adolescents differ from adults in multiple ways, some of which are relevant here. In particular, youth are in the process of physical and psychological development and have specific vulnerabilities depending upon where they are in this process. Second, they are dependent on their adult caregivers for their basic physical and emotional needs. Third, at least for those 4 years of age and older, their activities and social roles are largely centered around school, which can be a source of both great support and distress.

The first post-9/11 studies of adults reported that those living in the New York City (NYC) area and particularly those who directly witnessed the attack were most negatively affected [6–8]. For adults, the measure of their direct exposure, including being injured, seeing the towers burn or fall, seeing the planes hit, seeing bodies fall from the towers, being in or near the dust cloud, or being evacuated to safety became central to understanding subsequent mental health effects. Simultaneously, the initial studies investigating the effects of 9/11 on children living in NYC suggested similar results [9–11]. But it was quickly recognized that even children and adolescents not present at Ground Zero could be profoundly affected if family members were exposed, especially if exposure affected their functioning and parenting. This indirect exposure did not require the death or injury of a parent to have a negative effect. For example, if a child's home environment felt unsafe or insecure because of worry about a parents' well-being due to 9/11-related activities, such as being a first responder or having been evacuated from a WTC area building, that home and the child(ren) in it were essentially, indirectly 'infected' with 9/11 trauma. The safety of their lived environment was compromised after 9/11 for an extended period of time. Thus for research on children and adolescents, it became important to understand both direct exposure and different forms of indirect exposure, especially through family exposure.

Studies of Directly Exposed New York City Children and Adolescents

It has been estimated that 25,000 children were in close proximity to the WTC on 9/11 [12], and many child-focused studies explored the relationship between direct exposure and subsequent mental health outcomes. A study looking at early effects found that 1–2 months after September 11, 60% of parents in NYC reported that their children were upset by the attacks [8]. Similarly, a study of children living in NYC 4 months after 9/11 found that, according to parental reports, 18% had very high levels of PTSD symptoms, while another 66% had moderate PTSD symptoms [13]. A citywide investigation of 8236 NYC public school children, known as the World Trade Center-Board of Education (WTC-BOE) Study, examined a representative sample of NYC public school students in grades 4–12 using students' self-report rather than parental impressions and was conducted 6 months after 9/11. It found that 28.6% of the sample had probable anxiety or depressive disorders [10]. Another study of NYC school children, with high rates of pre-9/11 exposure to trauma, found that 2.5 years after the WTC attack, 35% met criteria for PTSD. In addition, almost half of these students could be classified as functionally impaired [11].

Moreover, direct or high-level exposure was identified by a number of studies as a particularly salient risk factor, establishing a dose-response relationship. For example, the WTC-BOE Study found that level of exposure was associated with high rates of probable disorders [10]: probable PTSD was 10.6% for the full sample but 18.4% for those with severe exposures. Similarly, for probable major depression, it was 8.1% (overall) and 11% (severe exposure), probable agoraphobia 14.8% (overall) and 21.8% (severe exposure), probable separation anxiety 12.3% (overall) and 20.1% (severe exposure), probable generalized anxiety disorder 10.3% (overall) and 14.1% (severe exposure), probable panic disorder 8.7% (overall) and 13.0% (severe exposure), and probable conduct disorder 12.8% (overall) and 14.3% (severe exposure). For those in grades 6–12, probable alcohol abuse/dependence was at 4.5% (overall) and 6.0% (severe exposure). These rates were up to three times higher compared with rates in same-aged youth pre-9/11 according to epidemiological studies [10].

A study investigating lower Manhattan pre-schoolers operationalized 'high-intensity' exposure as directly witnessing the towers collapsing, injured or dead people, or people jumping out of the towers. It was found that pre-schoolers who had witnessed at least one high-intensity exposure were nearly three times as likely to be either depressed or anxious and nearly five times as likely to have sleep problems [14]. Another study of lower Manhattan pre-schoolers similarly found that higher exposure was associated with more PTSD symptoms [9].

Direct exposure was also associated with an increased risk of behavioral problems among adolescents 6–7 years after 9/11, who were aged 5–12 at the time of the attack [5], as well as with an increased risk of substance use in these adolescents. Compared with adolescents who had not been exposed, those with one exposure-related risk factor were five times more likely to report substance use, those with two exposure-related risk factors had eight times greater risk, while those reporting three or more exposure-related risk factors had nearly 19 times increased risk of substance use [15].

A number of studies found that proximity to the WTC was associated with higher levels of symptoms (e.g. [13]). Interestingly, however, the WTC-BOE Study found that children attending schools very close to the WTC actually had lower rates of anxiety or depressive disorders compared with students attending school in other areas of New York City. The authors speculated that this might have been due to the high level of mental health and general support services that were specifically targeted at this population of youth in the immediate aftermath of the attacks [10].

In summary, these findings established that direct exposure to 9/11 as a child or adolescent resulted in elevated rates of a range of psychiatric and behavioural problems, not just PTSD, and that the outcomes showed a dose response to the intensity of exposure. These studies also illustrate gaps in the research approach. For example, exposure intensity was identified as being important yet was often measured by recall months after the event. It would be helpful to be prepared for the next disaster so that researchers could measure exposure as soon after a disaster as possible using self-report and possibly also other observational measures.

It would also be helpful to measure the effects of the exposure longitudinally, starting as early as possible. This might have documented, for example, that children nearest Ground Zero had high rates of distress soon after the disaster but that they were eased by services that were made available. While we conjecture this pattern, to be able to prove it would help the design of future interventions.

Family Exposure

Many children who did not live in the immediate vicinity of the WTC, and who therefore did not directly witness the attack, nevertheless had high levels of indirect exposure by having family members or friends who were in or near the WTC during the attack. Family exposure, defined as having a family member who was killed or injured or who was in or near the WTC at the time of the attack, was more strongly associated with psychopathology than direct exposure, in some studies [10]. A latent class analysis of the WTC-BOE data identified four classes of participants and found that indirect exposure was associated with membership in the class with the most severe profile of psychopathology and impairment [16]. As mentioned above, this may be understood as chronic exposure, in the home, to the effects of 9/11 through loss of a parent, dysfunction in a parent, illness in a parent, or unemployment of a parent, to name a few examples of 9/11 sequelae on families.

It has been estimated that more than 3250 children lost at least one parent in the attack [17]. Understandably, bereavement had a particularly strong impact on mental health, with significantly more bereaved children having at least one psychiatric disorder compared with non-bereaved children [18]. The differences were particularly remarkable for PTSD (29.6% bereaved vs 2.9% non-bereaved). Fortunately, the rates for all disorders declined for both groups over time. Another analysis of selected data from the WTC-BOE Study [10] found 16% of children who had a family member or friend who died in the attack screened positive for probable PTSD, compared with 7% of those who did not [19]. Another analysis reported PTSD rates of 17.6% among children who lost a family member in the attack [20]. In that analysis, an interaction effect was found among those who had both direct exposure and had a family member die in the attack, resulting in rates of 36.4% of probable PTSD.

There were, of course, many more children who were non-bereaved but whose parents were involved in 9/11 in some way, either by being present at Ground Zero, being evacuated from the WTC itself, or through their work as FRs, and these children and adolescents also showed significant psychological effects. As mentioned, the WTC-BOE Study found that the children and adolescents of WTC evacuees and FRs had even higher rates of mental health problems than directly exposed children and adolescents, as well as having elevated rates of substance use/abuse [10, 21, 22]. Researchers note that the mechanism by which parental trauma contributes to their offspring's psychopathology is unknown. However, the finding is of vital importance as this mode of transmission has not been a focus of post-disaster service intervention in the past.

The WTC-BOE Study also examined the differential impact of 9/11 on children of different types of FRs. The highest rate was among children of emergency medical technicians (18.9%), the next highest was among children of police officers (10.6%), and the lowest rate was found among children of firefighters (5.6%) [23]. The authors suggested that these differences could partially be explained by a combination of selective demographics of these professions, as well as rates of parental exposure. They also suggested that the appraisal of firefighters as 'heroes' may have been a factor that moderated distress among their children.

Kaitz et al. [24] reviewed several proposed mechanisms for the transmission of trauma, including parental distress, altered parenting behaviors, more general disturbances in parental thinking and behaviors, and growing up in a stressed household environment that may operate not only psychologically but biologically through cortisol and the HPA axis. Yehuda and Bierer [25] report that the transgenerational transmission of trauma has been described in a number of different types of parental trauma, ranging from combat to the Holocaust to sexual abuse. They argue that in addition to an environmental transmission, based on parents' behaviors, there may also be, for those born after the trauma, an epigenetic modality of transmission, in which a parent's epigenetic profile might be modified by trauma and/ or PTSD, and this modification passed along to offspring.

Yet another modality of transmission involves pregnant mothers exposed to a trauma. While not directly relevant to the central concern of this chapter, namely, the population of children and adolescents who were born prior to 9/11 and exposed between ages 0–18, the issues related to prenatal exposure are complex and might also include epigenetics and may prove important for a more complete understanding of the multifactorial transmission of trauma. A burgeoning body of literature does indicate that the effects of stress exposure on pregnant mothers can be passed onto fetuses. Studies have also indicated that pregnant mothers exposed to the WTC attack were more likely to have low birth weight babies [26], while lower cortisol levels were observed among babies born to mothers who developed PTSD in response to 9/11 while pregnant [27].

In summary, the findings on family transmissions of 9/11 trauma are extremely important for research into the effects of 9/11 on children and adolescents as well as a powerful validation of prior work on trauma transmission. These findings have public health consequence as well, as they identify a set of youth who were not directly exposed to 9/11 and may not have been targeted for surveillance and preventative interventions without these findings. At the same time, this research exposes important gaps in our understanding. The multiple mechanisms of this intergenerational transmission (behavioral, environmental, biological, and epigenetic) are poorly understood. We need longitudinal studies that assess the effects of trauma soon after exposure, examine the family and household structures in detail, and track how those structures are altered over time by a traumatic exposure of a parent. We also need studies that integrate biological, epigenetic, and behavioral approaches and are sensitive to developmental stage of the children and adolescents involved. Finally, we need more studies that directly assess the mental health effects on children who were in utero during the time of 9/11 and assess epigenetic transmission to progeny born years after a parental trauma exposure.

We also need studies that can capture the differences between first responder families, to ascertain what protective factors are acting in the homes of firefighters and how we can use those protective factors in all households. More generally, these findings indicate that we need more research into preventive approaches that take the whole family into account. For example, we still do not know if just treating the traumatized parent will block the transmission of trauma.

National Effects and the Relation to Media Exposure

The effects of 9/11 were also felt by children outside of New York City [28]. One nationally representative study conducted in the first few days after the attack found that over a third of parents reported that their children had at least one stress symptom and that nearly half had been worried about their own safety or that of their loved ones [29]. Another survey conducted 1–2 months after 9/11 found that nearly half of the parents living outside of the NYC or Washington DC reported that their children were distressed by the attacks [8]. A study of children living in Seattle, Washington, conducted 2–9 weeks after 9/11, found that 77% of children reported being worried, while 68% said that they were upset by reminders of the attack [30].

In a web-based survey of a national sample of adolescents, 60% of those not living in the vicinity of the WTC reported feeling that their own life or the life of someone close to them was in danger as a result of the attack. They also reported some initial stress symptoms; however, these were reduced to a low level 1 year after the attack [31]. A national, repeated, cross-sectional survey of adolescents living in cities throughout the United States found that adolescents interviewed in Fall 2001 had 35% higher odds of experiencing presleep worry compared with those interviewed in Fall 1998 [32].

A study conducted in California compared 227 adolescents surveyed 4 weeks after 9/11 with a comparable group of Californian teenagers who had been surveyed 4 and 2 years before the WTC attack. The study found that those surveyed after 9/11 perceived their risk of dying from a natural disaster to be higher than those interviewed before 9/11 [33]. A study of 171 Californian high school students conducted 2–5 months after 9/11 reported changes in their daily life activities and in PTSD symptoms related to the attack. However, these pre-post 9/11 differences were not found when the experience sampling methods were used to measure momentary mood reports in the same sample [34].

The national effects described above may have been a result of exposure to the highly repeated and very disturbing media images and reporting in the days and weeks following 9/11. Many schoolchildren were undoubtedly exposed, through TV, to shocking images of the WTC North Tower burning, only to be further shocked by the second plane hitting the other tower and the visuals of both the towers collapsing [35]. Furthermore, in the days and weeks following the attack, videos and images of the events were featured heavily in news reports and were widely available via the internet, causing many children and adolescents to be highly exposed to these images [36]. Nevertheless, the mental health consequence of exposure to distressing media images has been the subject of much debate [4].

Interestingly, among those living in NYC, more exposure to distressing media images was associated with more severe posttraumatic reactions in children [13] and adolescents [37]. However, analysis of the WTC-BOE data found that the association between intensive media use and PTSD was more likely to occur among those who were not directly exposed to the attacks [36]. Similarly, among elementary schoolchildren in Washington DC, who were not directly exposed, greater television exposure to the events of 9/11 was associated with increased distress [38]. Most importantly, studies conducted among children not living near NYC or Washington DC (both 9/11 attack sites) also reported an association between greater media exposure and increased symptoms of PTSD in children [29, 35].

In summary, the findings on the national effects of the local 9/11 attacks for both adults and children/adolescents are striking in that individuals thousands of miles from the trauma site were significantly psychologically impacted. The public health consequences are immense and run counter to traditional models of local emergency response. They have even affected the very definitions of PTSD in the DSM-5 [39]. At the same time, the mechanism of this traumatization at a distance remains unclear. Marshall et al. [40] put forth potential models that include the idea of shared 'ongoing threat' that may now apply, not only to terrorism but to the increasingly frequent and ubiquitous weather and earthquake phenomena. And, while it is seems hard to develop a model of the national effect that does not include media as a traumatic transmitter, the role of media remains controversial [41]. Thus we sorely need research that can clarify the role media plays in the immediate aftermath of a mass trauma, to discover ways of limiting the traumatic contagion. In particular, we need to understand whether and how the response to mass media depictions of trauma differs between children, adolescents, and adults. Intuitively, it seems that adolescents and especially children would have fewer defences than adults against disturbing images or the fear they elicit, but this will need to be explored. We also need far more in-depth and longitudinal research across wider geographic territory to understand the ancillary mechanism of this nationalization of a local trauma for children and adolescents, as well as research on how to curb those mechanisms once they are understood.

Risk and Resilience Factors

Prior Exposure to Traumatic Events and Violence

Prior trauma exposure was associated with a substantially increased risk for PTSD symptoms in pre-schoolers [9], as probable anxiety or depressive disorders in school-aged children [10], following 9/11. Prior trauma exposure was also found to increase the impact of high-intensity exposure to the WTC attack on child behavioral problems [14]. For NYC children with low prior exposure, a dose-response impact of the WTC attack was still evident 2.5 years after the attack [11]. In contrast, for those who had higher pre-attack trauma exposure, the severity of their post-traumatic distress 2.5 years later was best predicted by pre-9/11 trauma exposure, rather than the level of exposure on 9/11. In other words, prior trauma exposure was an important risk factor for subsequent distress and significantly compounded the effects of any exposure to 9/11. Pre-9/11 exposure to violence also emerged as a predictor of post-9/11 PTSD, depression, and conduct disorder symptoms, regardless of whether the exposure involved the adolescent as a witness or a victim of the violence [37].

Prior Mental Health Problems

Unfortunately, few studies investigated pre-9/11 mental health problems as risk factors for attack problems. However, a few ongoing longitudinal studies did include questions investigating the role of prior mental health as a predictor of distress following 9/11 [28]. Children who had exhibited higher levels of depression or anxiety 6 years prior to 9/11, when they were aged five, had higher levels of fear and anxiety in the months after the WTC attack [28]. Similarly, adolescents with a history of mental health problems were more distressed by the 9/11 events [34]. It should be noted, however, that one study did not find any moderation effect of prior mental health symptoms on the relationship between exposure to 9/11 and subsequent mental health symptom level [37].

Parental Reactions

In addition to parents' ability to transmit trauma to their unexposed children and adolescents, a number of studies indicate that parental reactions may have mediated or moderated their exposed child's reactions to 9/11. Parents reporting substantial stress symptoms in the days after the attack were more than twice as likely to report that their children had stress symptoms [29], while children whose parents had possible PTSD were found to be over four times more likely to have severe PTSD symptoms themselves [13]. Children living in NYC who saw their parents crying following the attack were also more than three times more likely to have severe PTSD symptoms than those who did not [13], and NYC adolescents who saw a parent crying were more likely to have behaviour problems 6 months after the attack compared with other adolescents [42]. It should be noted, however, that the aforementioned studies were based on parental reports which may bias the findings.

Nevertheless, other studies that did not rely on parental report reinforce the finding that parental reactions had an impact on their child's mental health response to 9/11. For example, there is evidence from a study of Lower Manhattan pre-schoolers that young children of mothers with co-occurring probable PTSD and depression were independently rated as having more behaviour problems by their teachers, compared with mothers with depression only or with neither disorder, 2–4 years after the attack [43]. A study conducted in Washington DC showed that parents with more distress were more likely to report distress among their children, but this was consistent with the children's self-report of their own distress [30]. Finally, two adolescent studies showed that parental distress or endorsement of PTSD symptoms was associated with their teenage children's PTSD symptoms [44] and behavioral difficulties [5]. These findings indicate that parental reactions likely played an important role in moderating or mediating offspring's responses to 9/11 and were not merely the result of biased ratings provided by distressed parents. This raises a question about mechanisms. Were these children/adolescents more distressed because they had been 'infected' by their parents' traumatic reactions, or does this reflect a more general family vulnerability for distress reactions due to biological, economic, and social risk factors affecting both parent and child? Again, the answer to this question would help direct interventions more effectively.

Economic Resources

The 9/11 attack impacted the economic stability of the United States, and many youths, most especially in NYC, found themselves affected financially. For example, in a study of high school students in Bronx County 8 months after the event, participants who reported financial difficulty as a result of the attack were five times more likely to have PTSD [45]. Many people living in the NYC area lost their jobs as a result of the attack [46], and studies investigating the impact of this on child mental health found that parental job loss was associated with higher levels of PTSD and other anxiety disorders [46], as well as being significantly associated with parental PTSD and depression [53], which in turn was associated with child anxiety and poor family relationships.

In summary, research on risk factors for mental health sequelae to 9/11 exposure have begun to identify individual, family, and contextual economic factors that predispose children/adolescents to the development of negative outcomes and could potentially serve as targets for preventive interventions. Yet these risk factors also raise many questions for public health research and intervention. Should we, for example, identify children/adolescents with prior trauma or mental health conditions for special intervention after a mass trauma? Should those treating these individuals be especially vigilant in monitoring these individuals after a mass trauma? How can we transform prior challenges into resilience-building experiences rather than deficits? Can parents be trained to respond to mass traumas in ways that are less damaging to their children? Is economic recovery a public health concern? To answer these questions will require the type of research we have been advocating throughout this chapter. We will need research that includes large representative samples with appropriate controls, the use of in-depth assessments across multiple biopsychosocial domains, a developmentally oriented longitudinal design, and timely initiation after a trauma.

Health Care Utilization by Children/Adolescents Affected by 9/11

The evidence in the studies reviewed here indicates that there was a significant mental health impact on children and adolescents from exposure to 9/11, particularly among those directly exposed or who were indirectly exposed through their families. This further suggests that there was also a significant need for mental health services to provide support and treatment for young people who were affected. Thus, an additional area of public health interest is to determine if these services were sought and how well the mental health needs were met by existing delivery systems.

Based on the WTC-BOE data, there is evidence that around 18% of children living in NYC utilized mental health services in the months following the attacks, with more than half of those receiving support services in school [49]. There was a 24% rate of mental health service use among children who were directly exposed and a 30% rate of use among those meeting criteria for probable PTSD. While this indicates that mental health service use was more likely to be provided to those in need, it still highlights the large numbers of children who met criteria for a probable disorder, yet had not sought out mental health treatment, and perhaps were not even aware of services that were and continue to be available for this population [54]. This suggests a need for greater outreach in the wake of such a disaster, perhaps school-wide interventions, and not limited to those in the immediate proximity of the event.

It should be noted, however, that those living in the immediate vicinity of the WTC attack and who were exposed to the dust cloud that was generated when the towers fell were also most likely to be at increased risk for a range of physical health problems, such as respiratory problems, gastrointestinal symptoms, allergies, and cancer, among others [48, 51, 54]. Moreover, physical health problems are risk factors for mental health problems and vice versa. These potential interactions can be seen, for example, in a cross-sectional study conducted among adolescents with asthma 10–11 years after 9/11, who had been in close proximity to the WTC at the time of the attack. The study found that probable PTSD was associated with poorly controlled asthma [12]. It is, therefore, important to think about both traumatic and toxic exposures, both physical health problems and mental health problems as all part of an interacting system, in which comorbidities are common and mutually reinforcing.

Individuals suffering mental health problems as a result of their exposure to 9/11 are now known to be at increased likelihood of presenting to primary care physicians [50, 52]. Primary care physicians working in the NYC area should consider asking their patients whether they were exposed to the attacks, and what the nature of their exposure was, as this information may help them to better diagnose and treat their patients with both physical and mental disorders. In this respect, the NYC Department of Health have developed a set of clinical guidelines for physicians that clarify potential reactions to 9/11 among children and adolescents and include treatment recommendations [47].

In summary, from a population perspective, we know very little about the unmet mental and physical health care needs of children/adolescents exposed to 9/11. While we are gaining knowledge about their physical and mental health outcomes despite the small and generally unrepresentative samples, we know less about service utilization and its effectiveness. One barrier to research has been that the services that are accessed are distributed across a complex health care system with poor central communication. Nevertheless, we need to find creative ways to answer these questions, so we might better serve those already suffering from 9/11-related traumatic exposures as children and adolescents, as well as those who will become exposed to other mass traumas in the future.

Conclusions

In each of the sections above, we attempted to summarize the most relevant findings, as well as critique limitations of the existing relevant research, and to make recommendations for future investigations. We conclude with an overview of what we have learned, what we have missed, and how we might better proceed in the future to protect our most vulnerable and most precious citizens, our youth, in the face of mass trauma.

What emerges from the literature is that many individuals throughout the United States who were children or adolescents on 9/11 were and continue to be profoundly affected in a myriad of ways as a result of that event. Not surprisingly, distress was highest among children and adolescents who lived in close proximity to the WTC and were either exposed directly or were living away from Ground Zero but were indirectly exposed through their families. For many living outside of New York with neither direct nor indirect exposure, the attack impacted their sense of safety and well-being nevertheless, and some developed mental health symptoms in reaction to the attack, particularly those with greater media exposure. Having prior trauma or mental health issues and having a parent who developed PTSD or other distress were associated with higher levels of child mental health problems. Low socio-economic status and life disruptions resulting from 9/11, including parental job loss and physical health problems, also compounded the distress of children and adolescents. Comorbidities between traumatic exposures and toxic exposures on and immediately following 9/11, as well as other physical-mental health comorbidities, are just beginning to be recognized in those exposed during childhood or adolescence and who are now entering young adulthood or are already into the third decade of life. Although many have utilized mental health services, there clearly remains a large unmet need for mental and physical health services that are appropriately targeted and effective.

The existing body of research has significant limitations, partly because a focus on children/adolescents was possibly viewed as less important than on adults, many of whom died. Many research studies did not begin immediately after 9/11, as would have been ideal, and subsequently, much of it was conducted within 2 years of the disaster and then stopped. Consequently, much of the research has been too little, too late, without planned follow-up, insufficiently powered samples, and with almost a total lack of valid comparison groups. Most importantly, we cannot learn from information never collected.

We need to proceed based on a life course perspective that recognizes that childhood is a vulnerable, developmental period and that well-being during childhood often determines successful educational, occupational, and social functioning into adulthood. Individual development takes place in a context that influences how children process their experiences, and, therefore, understanding the consequences of events in childhood requires repeated contextual, physical, and psychosocial assessments that are sensitive to developmental phases across the life course.

Based on these principles, we advocate for research that contains meaningful representative samples with matched controls and that is longitudinal in design and developmentally focused. The research needs to be based on the best practice of epidemiologic research in terms of field-based, face-to-face evaluations with multiple informants and valid, reliable measures of mental health symptoms and conditions, as well as of other key constructs. These studies must include comprehensive biopsychosocial assessments that address the crucial factors that the existing literature has identified as important, such as neighbourhood characteristics; school characteristics; family context; parenting styles before and after the event; prior mental, physical, and learning challenges; in-depth assessment as to the nature of the exposure; and thorough assessment of physical, psychiatric, behavioral, and role-functioning outcomes. To capture the interface biologically and psychologically, we will need to conduct thorough physical assessments and to collect key biomarkers such as genetics, epigenetics, inflammatory signals, and stress-related hormones, as well as a judicious use of neuroimaging.

While this is a formidable challenge, the closer we come to achieving it, the better we will be prepared to support the next generation as it faces the challenges of past and future trauma.

References

1. Klassen TP, Hartling L, Craig JC, Offringa M. Children are not just small adults: the urgent need for high-quality trial evidence in children. PLoS Med. 2008;5(8):e172.
2. Eisenberg N, Silver RC. Growing up in the shadow of terrorism: youth in America after 9/11. Am Psychol. 2011;66(6):468.
3. Rousseau C, Jamil U, Bhui K, Boudjarane M. Consequences of 9/11 and the war on terror on children's and young adult's mental health: a systematic review of the past 10 years. Clin Child Psychol Psychiatry. 2015;20(2):173–93.
4. Gershoff ET, Aber JL. Editors' Introduction: assessing the impact of September 11th, 2001, on children, youth, and parents: methodological challenges to research on terrorism and other nonnormative events. Appl Dev Sci. 2004;8(3):106–10.
5. Mann M, Li J, Farfel MR, Maslow CB, Osahan S, Stellman SD. Adolescent behavior and PTSD 6–7 years after the World Trade Center terrorist attacks of September 11, 2001. Disaster Health. 2014;2(3-4):121–9. doi:10.1080/21665044.2015.1010931.

6. DiGrande L, Perrin MA, Thorpe LE, Thalji L, Murphy J, Wu D, Farfel M, Brackbill RM. Posttraumatic stress symptoms, PTSD, and risk factors among lower Manhattan residents 2–3 years after the September 11, 2001 terrorist attacks. J Traum Stress. 2008;21(3):264–73.
7. Galea S, Ahern J, Resnick H, Kilpatrick D, Bucuvalas M, Gold J, Vlahov D. Psychological sequelae of the September 11 terrorist attacks in New York City. N Engl J Med. 2002;346(13):982–7.
8. Schlenger WE, Caddell JM, Ebert L, Jordan BK, Rourke KM, Wilson D, Thalji L, Dennis JM, Fairbank JA, Kulka RA. Psychological reactions to terrorist attacks: findings from the National Study of Americans' Reactions to September 11. Jama. 2002;288(5):581–8.
9. DeVoe ER, Klein TP, Bannon W Jr, Miranda-Julian C. Young children in the aftermath of the World Trade Center attacks. Psychol Trauma Theory Res Pract Policy. 2011;3(1):1.
10. Hoven CW, Duarte CS, Lucas CP, Wu P, Mandell DJ, Goodwin RD, Cohen M, Balaban V, Woodruff BA, Bin F. Psychopathology among New York City public school children 6 months after September 11. Arch Gen Psychiatry. 2005;62(5):545–51.
11. Mullett-Hume E, Anshel D, Guevara V, Cloitre M. Cumulative trauma and posttraumatic stress disorder among children exposed to the 9/11 World Trade Center attack. Am J Orthopsychiatry. 2008;78(1):103.
12. Gargano LM, Thomas PA, Stellman SD. Asthma control in adolescents 10 to 11 y after exposure to the World Trade Center disaster. Pediatr Res. 2016;81(1–1):43–50. doi:10.1038/pr.2016.190.
13. Fairbrother G, Stuber J, Galea S, Fleischman AR, Pfefferbaum B. Posttraumatic stress reactions in New York City children after the September 11, 2001, terrorist attacks. Ambul Pediatr. 2003;3(6):304–11. doi:10.1367/1539-4409(2003)003<0304:PSRINY>2.0.CO;2.
14. Chemtob CM, Nomura Y, Abramovitz RA. Impact of conjoined exposure to the World Trade Center attacks and to other traumatic events on the behavioral problems of preschool children. Arch Pediatr Adolesc Med. 2008;162(2):126–33.
15. Chemtob C, Nomura Y, Josephson L, Adams RE, Sederer L. Substance use and functional impairment among adolescents directly exposed to the 2001 World Trade Center attacks. Disasters. 2009;33(3):337–52.
16. Alman LG, Guffanti G, Fan B, Duarte C, Wu P, Musa G, Cohen P, Poli M, Hoven C. O-15-Latent class analysis of ptsd symptoms among 6733 New York City students exposed to 9/11. Eur Psychiatry. 2012;27:1.
17. Coates SW, Schechter DS, First E. Brief interventions with traumatized children and families after September 11. In: Trauma and human bonds. Hillsdale, NJ: Analytic; 2003.
18. Pfeffer CR, Altemus M, Heo M, Jiang H. Salivary cortisol and psychopathology in children bereaved by the September 11, 2001 terror attacks. Biol Psychiatry. 2007;61(8):957–65.
19. Rosen CS, Cohen M. Subgroups of New York City children at high risk of PTSD after the September 11 attacks: a signal detection analysis. Psychiatr Serv. 2010;61(1):64–9.
20. Hoven CW, Duarte CS, Wu P, Doan T, Singh N, Mandell DJ, Bin F, Teichman Y, Teichman M, Wicks J. Parental exposure to mass violence and child mental health: the first responder and WTC evacuee study. Clin Child Fam Psychol Rev. 2009;12(2):95–112.
21. Hoven CW, Duarte CS, Wu P, Erickson EA, Musa GJ, Mandell DJ. Exposure to trauma and separation anxiety in children after the WTC attack. Appl Dev Sci. 2004;8(4):172–83.
22. Wu P, Duarte CS, Mandell DJ, Fan B, Liu X, Fuller CJ, Musa G, Cohen M, Cohen P, Hoven CW. Exposure to the World Trade Center attack and the use of cigarettes and alcohol among New York City public high-school students. Am J Public Health. 2006;96(5):804–7.
23. Duarte CS, Hoven CW, Wu P, Bin F, Cotel S, Mandell DJ, Nagasawa M, Balaban V, Wernikoff L, Markenson D. Posttraumatic stress in children with first responders in their families. J Trauma Stress. 2006;19(2):301–6.
24. Kaitz M, Levy M, Ebstein R, Faraone SV, Mankuta D. The intergenerational effects of trauma from terror: a real possibility. Infant Ment Health J. 2009;30(2):158–79.
25. Yehuda R, Bierer LM. Transgenerational transmission of cortisol and PTSD risk. Prog Brain Res. 2007;167:121–35.

26. Berkowitz GS, Wolff MS, Janevic TM, Holzman IR, Yehuda R, Landrigan PJ. The World Trade Center disaster and intrauterine growth restriction. Jama. 2003;290(5):595–6.

27. Yehuda R, Engel SM, Brand SR, Seckl J, Marcus SM, Berkowitz GS. Transgenerational effects of posttraumatic stress disorder in babies of mothers exposed to the World Trade Center attacks during pregnancy. J Clin Endocrinol Metab. 2005;90(7):4115–8.

28. Hock E, Hart M, Kang MJ, Lutz WJ. Predicting children's reactions to terrorist attacks: the importance of self-reports and preexisting characteristics. Am J Orthopsychiatry. 2004;74(3):253.

29. Schuster MA, Stein BD, Jaycox LH, Collins RL, Marshall GN, Elliott MN, Zhou AJ, Kanouse DE, Morrison JL, Berry SH. A national survey of stress reactions after the September 11, 2001, terrorist attacks. N Engl J Med. 2001;345(20):1507–12. doi:10.1056/NEJM200111153452024.

30. Lengua LJ, Long AC, Smith KI, Meltzoff AN. Pre-attack symptomatology and temperament as predictors of children's responses to the September 11 terrorist attacks. J Child Psychol Psychiatry. 2005;46(6):631–45.

31. Gil-Rivas V, Holman EA, Silver RC. Adolescent vulnerability following the September 11th terrorist attacks: a study of parents and their children. Appl Dev Sci. 2004;8(3):130–42.

32. Mijanovich T, Weitzman BC. Disaster in context: the effects of 9/11 on youth distant from the attacks. Community Ment Health J. 2010;46(6):601–11.

33. Halpern-Felsher BL, Millstein SG. The effects of terrorism on teens' perceptions of dying: the new world is riskier than ever. J Adolesc Health. 2002;30(5):308–11.

34. Whalen CK, Henker B, King PS, Jamner LD, Levine L. Adolescents react to the events of September 11, 2001: focused versus ambient impact. J Abnorm Child Psychol. 2004;32(1):1–11.

35. Saylor CF, Cowart BL, Lipovsky JA, Jackson C, Finch A. Media exposure to September 11 elementary school students' experiences and posttraumatic symptoms. Am Behav Sci. 2003;46(12):1622–42.

36. Duarte CS, Wu P, Cheung A, Mandell DJ, Fan B, Wicks J, Musa GJ, Hoven CW. Media use by children and adolescents from New York City 6 months after the WTC attack. J Trauma Stress. 2011;24(5):553–6.

37. Aber JL, Gershoff ET, Ware A, Kotler JA. Estimating the effects of September 11th and other forms of violence on the mental health and social development of New York City's youth: a matter of context. Appl Dev Sci. 2004;8(3):111–29. doi:10.1207/s1532480xads0803_2.

38. Phillips D, Prince S, Schiebelhut L. Elementary school children's responses 3 months after the September 11 terrorist attacks: a study in Washington, DC. Am J Orthopsychiatry. 2004;74(4):509.

39. Friedman MJ, Resick PA, Bryant RA, Brewin CR. Considering PTSD for DSM-5. Depress Anxiety. 2011;28(9):750–69.

40. Marshall RD, Bryant RA, Amsel L, Suh EJ, Cook JM, Neria Y. The psychology of ongoing threat: relative risk appraisal, the September 11 attacks, and terrorism-related fears. Am Psychol. 2007;62(4):304.

41. Weidmann A, Papsdorf J. Witnessing trauma in the newsroom: posttraumatic symptoms in television journalists exposed to violent news clips. J Nerv Ment Dis. 2010;198(4):264–71.

42. Stuber J, Galea S, Pfefferbaum B, Vandivere S, Moore K, Fairbrother G. Behavior problems in New York City's children after the September 11, 2001, terrorist attacks. Am J Orthopsychiatry. 2005;75(2):190.

43. Chemtob CM, Nomura Y, Rajendran K, Yehuda R, Schwartz D, Abramovitz R. Impact of maternal posttraumatic stress disorder and depression following exposure to the September 11 attacks on preschool children's behavior. Child Dev. 2010;81(4):1129–41.

44. Gil Rivas V, Silver RC, Holman EA, McIntosh DN, Poulin M. Parental response and adolescent adjustment to the September 11, 2001 terrorist attacks. J Traum Stress. 2007;20(6):1063–8.

45. Calderoni ME, Alderman EM, Silver EJ, Bauman LJ. The mental health impact of 9/11 on inner-city high school students 20 miles north of Ground Zero. J Adolesc Health. 2006;39(1):57–65.

46. Comer JS, Fan B, Duarte CS, Wu P, Musa GJ, Mandell DJ, Albano AM, Hoven CW. Attack-related life disruption and child psychopathology in New York City public schoolchildren

6-months post-9/11. J Clin Child Adolesc Psychol. 2010;39(4):460–9. doi:10.1080/15374416. 2010.486314.

47. Cone J, Perlman S, Eros-Sarnyai M, Hoven C, Graber N, Galvez M, Fierman A, Kyvelos E, Thomas P. Clinical guidelines for children and adolescents exposed to the World Trade Center disaster City Health Information, vol. 28. New York, NY: New York City Department of Health and Mental Hygiene; 2009. p. 29–40.

48. Farfel M, DiGrande L, Brackbill R, Prann A, Cone J, Friedman S, Walker DJ, Pezeshki G, Thomas P, Galea S. An overview of 9/11 experiences and respiratory and mental health conditions among World Trade Center Health Registry enrollees. J Urban Health. 2008;85(6):880–909.

49. Graeff-Martins AS, Hoven CW, Wu P, Bin F, Duarte CS. Use of mental health services by children and adolescents six months after the world trade center attack. Psychiatr Serv. 2014;65(2):263–5.

50. Greene T, Neria Y, Gross R. Prevalence, detection and correlates of PTSD in the primary care setting: a systematic review. J Clin Psychol Med Settings. 2016;23(1):1–21.

51. Li J, Brackbill RM, Stellman SD, Farfel MR, Miller-Archie SA, Friedman S, Walker DJ, Thorpe LE, Cone J. Gastroesophageal reflux symptoms and comorbid asthma and posttraumatic stress disorder following the 9/11 terrorist attacks on World Trade Center in New York City. Am J Gastroenterol. 2011;106(11):1933–41.

52. Neria Y, Olfson M, Gameroff MJ, Wickramaratne P, Gross R, Pilowsky DJ, Blanco C, Manetti-Cusa J, Lantigua R, Shea S. The mental health consequences of disaster-related loss: findings from primary care one year after the 9/11 terrorist attacks. Psychiatry. 2008;71(4):339–48.

53. Ryan M, Wu P, Bin F, Shen S, Duarte C, Mus G, Chesaniuk M, Hoven C. Job loss related to 9/11 and child mental health. In: Paper presented at the Hunter College Psychology Conference, New York, NY, April 2014.

54. Welch AE, Caramanica K, Debchoudhury I, Pulizzi A, Farfel MR, Stellman SD, Cone JE. A qualitative examination of health and health care utilization after the September 11th terror attacks among World Trade Center Health Registry enrollees. BMC Public Health. 2012;12(1):1.

World Trade Center Related Health Among NYC Firefighters and EMS Workers

Jennifer Yip, Mayris P. Webber, Rachel Zeig-Owens, Madeline Vossbrinck, Ankura Singh, Theresa Schwartz, and David J. Prezant

Introduction

FDNY WTC Health Program: 2001–2016

On September 11, 2001 (9/11), the collapse of the World Trade Center (WTC) resulted in the loss of 343 Fire Department of the City of New York (FDNY) responders and exposed thousands more to a hazardous mix of inorganic dust, products of combustion and respirable particulates [1]. In response, FDNY Bureau of Health Services (FDNY-BHS) instituted a rigorous medical monitoring and treatment program for the nearly 16,000 FDNY firefighters and emergency medical service (EMS) workers who performed rescue/recovery work on 9/11 and during the subsequent 10-month recovery period at the WTC site. Concurrently, FDNY physicians and others documented the early health symptoms and conditions presented by the FDNY workforce, most notably respiratory and mental health symptoms, which were the most problematic immediately post-disaster. In 2005, the FDNY data center was established to institutionalize the collection and analysis of data on health conditions associated with WTC exposure.

J. Yip • R. Zeig-Owens • M. Vossbrinck • A. Singh
T. Schwartz • D.J. Prezant (✉)
Fire Department of the City of New York, Bureau of Health Services, 9 Metrotech Center, Brooklyn, New York, USA
e-mail: David.Prezant@fdny.nyc.gov

M.P. Webber
Department of Epidemiology and Population Health, Montefiore Medical Center and Albert Einstein College of Medicine, Bronx, New York, USA

Fire Department of the City of New York, Bureau of Health Services, 9 Metrotech Center, Brooklyn, New York, USA

© Springer International Publishing AG 2018   137
A.M. Szema (ed.), *World Trade Center Pulmonary Diseases and Multi-Organ System Manifestations*, DOI 10.1007/978-3-319-59372-2_10

FDNY's multifaceted approach (monitoring, treatment, and research) has enabled us to document and ameliorate the health effects of 9/11. FDNY-BHS and its WTC Health Program (WTCHP) provided clinical care and referrals for services, while research studies from the FDNY data center identified trends and risk factors for WTC-related health conditions to improve our understanding of exposure-host interactions and, in so doing, to provide appropriate clinical services. In this report, which is an update from a previous review article [2], we describe FDNY's post-9/11 clinical care and health interventions and provide a summary of health outcomes that we have identified between 2001 and 2016.

Evolution of the FDNY WTC Health Program

FDNY's WTC treatment program began on 9/11, when FDNY-BHS physicians were deployed to the WTC site, some prior to the collapse, to provide triage and on-site treatment. Treatment continued and three weeks after 9/11, formal medical monitoring began, leveraging the existing health infrastructure already in place at FDNY-BHS at the time of the disaster. This occupational health service was established well before 9/11 to provide monitoring and treatment medical exams for active FDNY firefighters and EMS workers, primarily to assess and improve their fitness to perform work-related activities. The early WTCHP incorporated FDNY-BHS routine exams that included physical examinations by FDNY physicians, self-administered health questionnaires (rapidly updated to include WTC-related questions), pulmonary function tests, chest x-rays, cardiograms, audiograms, and the collection of blood and urine samples for testing. Since then, the WTCHP, based in Brooklyn, NY, has added satellite locations in Queens, NY, Staten Island, NY, and Suffolk and Orange counties to increase access to care. It has also expanded to include more in-depth clinical exams and physical and mental health monitoring exams as well as free treatment services.

Free treatment services for WTC-related health conditions are offered to all active and retired WTC-exposed FDNY responders. FDNY-WTCHP provides on-site diagnosis and treatment of WTC-related physical health conditions (e.g., lower and upper respiratory diseases and gastroesophageal reflux disease [GERD]), mental health conditions (post-traumatic stress disorder [PTSD], depression, anxiety, prolonged grief, and substance abuse [primarily alcohol and tobacco use]), and when necessary referrals to an extensive network of specialty providers conveniently located in the New York metropolitan area. Referrals are provided for diagnostic procedures and treatment. After epidemiological findings from FDNY and others demonstrating a link between WTC exposure and cancer [3–5], and the subsequent addition of cancers as a WTC-covered condition in 2012 under the James Zadroga 9/11 Health and Compensation Act of 2010 Act [6], FDNY-WTCHP expanded to provide diagnostic evaluations for WTC-related cancers and added providers such as the Memorial Sloan Kettering Cancer Center to its external network for cancer treatment. Program expansion also included adding an FDNY case management unit primarily to provide care coordination for patients with cancer and other severe diseases, cancer screening for early diagnosis, and, for patients unresponsive to treatment, end-of-life care through hospice referrals.

WTC Health Program Utilization

There are 15,634 FDNY WTC-exposed responders enrolled in the FDNY-WTCHP. Since the inception of FDNY-WTCHP, 15,245 (98%) received at least one monitoring exam, and to date (December 1, 2016), 10,971 (70%) have received at least eight monitoring exams. Participation rates remain high; in the last 12 months, 10,818 (69%) enrolled members received an FDNY WTC monitoring exam.

Between 9/11 and 12/1/2016, not including monitoring, 14,028 (90%) individuals visited an FDNY-WTCHP physician for diagnosis and treatment of a physical health problem. Many of these conditions, initially acute, have evolved to become chronic illnesses requiring ongoing treatment. To date, 10,433 persons have been certified by the National Institute for Occupational Safety and Health (NIOSH) as having at least one WTC-related health condition, and 9484 (61% of enrolled members) have filled at least one medication under this program (Table 1). Over the last 12 months, 7718 (49%) enrolled members with at least one certified WTC-related illness have presented for treatment of a physical or mental health problem at the FDNY-WTCHP. The most common types of medications for physical health conditions were proton pump inhibitors for those certified with GERD; saline wash and nasal anti-inflammatory steroids for those certified with upper airway diseases, predominantly chronic rhinosinusitis (CRS); and beta-adrenergic agents and inhaled

Table 1 Selected characteristics of WTC-exposed firefighters and EMS workers enrolled in the FDNY World Trade Center Health Program[a]

Characteristics	Firefighters		EMS workers		Total	
	N	%	N	%	N	%
Total	13195	100	2439	100	15634	100
WTC arrival group						
Arrival on the morning of 9/11	1812	13.7	459	18.8	2271	14.5
Arrival during the afternoon of 9/11	6094	46.2	719	29.5	6813	43.6
Arrival on 9/12/2001	2442	18.5	293	12.0	2735	17.5
Arrival any day between 9/13/2001 and 9/24/2001	2042	15.5	603	24.7	2645	16.9
Arrival after 9/24/2001	265	2.0	215	8.8	480	3.1
Undefined exposure	540	4.1	150	6.2	690	4.4
Duration—months at the WTC						
Median [IQR range]	3 [1–5]		2 [1–5]		2 [1–5]	
Age on 9/11 years						
Median [IQR range]	40.6 [34.0–46.7]		34.9 [28.2–41.0]		39.6 [33.0–46.0]	
Gender						
Male	13165	99.8	1956	80.2	15121	96.7
Female	30	0.2	483	19.8	513	3.3
Race						
White	12340	93.5	1267	52.0	13607	87.0
Nonwhite	855	6.5	1172	48.1	2027	13.0

(continued)

Table 1 (continued)

Characteristics	Firefighters		EMS workers		Total	
	N	%	N	%	N	%
Total	13195	100	2439	100	15634	100
Current smoking status[a,b]						
Current	652	4.9	319	13.1	971	6.2
Former	4580	34.7	895	36.7	5475	35.0
Never	7680	58.2	1189	48.8	8869	56.7
Retirement status[a]						
Retired	8735	66.2	1304	53.5	10039	64.2
Not retired	4460	33.8	1135	46.5	5595	35.8
Post-9/11 prevalence of respiratory health diagnoses[c]						
Chronic rhinosinusitis	4618	35.0	357	14.6	4975	31.8
Gastroesophageal reflux disease	4396	33.3	379	15.5	4775	30.5
Obstructive airways disease	3733	28.3	334	13.7	4067	26.0
Asthma	2920	22.1	274	11.2	3194	20.4
Chronic bronchitis	1408	10.7	88	3.6	1496	9.6
Chronic obstructive pulmonary disease	256	1.9	19	0.8	275	1.8
At least one of the above respiratory diagnoses[c]	7202	54.6	665	27.3	7867	50.3
Prevalence of probable mental health conditions in year 15[d]						
PTSD	720	8.0	100	6.8	820	7.8
Depression	1395	15.4	223	15.1	1618	15.4
At least one medication fill under FDNY-WTCHP	8617	65.3	867	35.5	9484	60.6

[a]As of December 1, 2016
[b]$N = 319$ had unknown current smoking status
[c]Between 2001 and 2016
[d]Percentages of $N = 10,538$ who completed a mental health questionnaire in 9/11 year, year 15

corticosteroids for those certified with obstructive airways diseases (OAD) including asthma, reactive airways dysfunction syndrome (RADS), chronic bronchitis, and emphysema. The three most common types of medications for those certified with mental health conditions, predominantly PTSD, depression, and anxiety were selective serotonin reuptake inhibitors, anti-anxiety drugs, and norepinephrine and dopamine reuptake inhibitors.

WTC exposure

We use two measures to characterize WTC-exposure in our research studies: initial arrival time and duration of work at the WTC site. Initial arrival time was obtained from the earliest post-9/11 questionnaire, which was completed a median of four months after 9/11. Initial arrival time is categorized from highly exposed to least exposed as follows: arriving on the morning of 9/11 (highest exposure level); arriving during the afternoon of 9/11; arriving on 9/12/2001; arriving any day between 9/13/2001 and 9/24/2001; and arriving after 9/24/2001 (lowest exposure level). Duration of work was added to later questionnaires and was obtained a median of four years post-9/11. Duration of work is a summation of each calendar month that an individual worked for at least one day at the WTC site (range 1–10 months). For most analyses, we did not have a non-WTC-exposed group, as virtually all active FDNY members worked at the WTC site. Table 1 shows that close to 14% of firefighters and 19% of EMS workers arrived at the WTC site during the morning of 9/11, although most firefighters (46%) and EMS workers (30%) arrived during that afternoon. The median duration of time worked at the site was three months for firefighters and two months for EMS workers. The FDNY-WTC rescue/recovery cohort was mostly white (87%), was male (97%), and had a median age of 40 years (IQR range: 33–46 years) on 9/11.

WTC Health Findings

To describe various health conditions, we use both self-reported symptoms from monitoring questionnaires and physician diagnoses from FDNY medical records. Pulmonary function was analyzed using forced vital capacity (FVC) and the forced expiratory volume in the first second (FEV$_1$) results from routine spirometry. Bronchial reactivity information was obtained from methacholine challenge tests.

Pulmonary Function and Lower Respiratory

Among 12,781 WTC-exposed firefighters and EMS workers who had 61,746 spirometry measurements, [7] reported accelerated lung function decline from serial FEV$_1$ measurements, which averaged 372 ml over the first year after 9/11, the equivalent of 10–12 years of normal, age-related loss. During the subsequent six years post-disaster, there was little to no recovery. In updated studies extending follow-up time up to 14 years after 9/11, most firefighters and EMS workers continued to show a lack of lung function recovery [8, 9]. The dose-response association of WTC exposure in relation to lung function remained: firefighters who arrived during the morning of 9/11 averaged lower lung function than did lesser exposed firefighters, a difference that remained statistically significant during most of the follow-up [10].

Methacholine challenge tests identify individuals with bronchial hyperreactivity (BHR), a hallmark of asthma/RADS. At six months post-9/11, firefighters who arrived during the morning of 9/11 were 6.8 times more likely to experience BHR than those who arrived later (odds ratio [OR]: 6.8; 95% CI: 1.8–25.2) [11]. Further, in a recent follow-up study, we found that for many, BHR did not resolve with removal from the noxious exposure, even more than one decade post-9/11, and that persistent BHR predicted an accelerated decline in lung function [10].

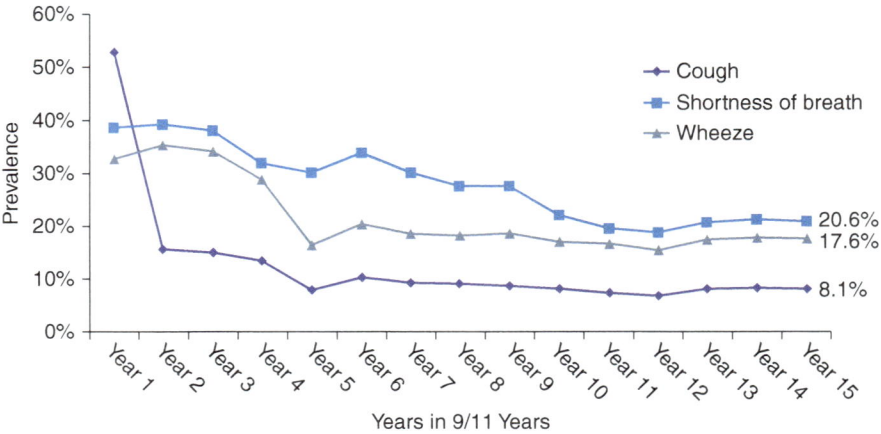

Fig. 1 Prevalence of lower respiratory symptoms by FDNY-WTC responders

Figure 1 shows that immediately after 9/11, cough was the most common respiratory symptom reported by 53% of the FDNY-WTC rescue/recovery cohort, followed by shortness of breath (38%) and wheezing (33%). In the first published post-9/11 study on respiratory health, [1] described "World Trade Center cough syndrome" in an initial sample of 332 WTC-exposed firefighters who were evaluated 6 months after 9/11. WTC cough syndrome was characterized by a constellation of symptoms including a persistent cough and upper respiratory and lower respiratory symptoms (e.g., nasal congestion, nasal drip, sore throat, bronchial hyperreactivity, and/or GERD symptoms). In this sample of 332, the prevalence of this syndrome was greatest in those arriving earliest at the WTC site, on the morning of 9/11 [1].

Subsequent studies confirmed the association between WTC-exposure intensity (as measured by arrival time) and lower respiratory conditions, such as OAD. OAD includes the following physician diagnoses from FDNY medical records: asthma/RADS, chronic obstructive pulmonary disease/emphysema, and chronic bronchitis. In a sample of 8930 firefighters, those who arrived during the morning of 9/11 had four times the OAD diagnosis rate (relative rate, 3.96; 95% CI, 2.51–6.26) of later-arriving firefighters during the first 15 months after 9/11 [12]. Similarly, EMS workers with the earliest arrival time have more than twice the risk (relative risk, 2.4; 95% CI, 1.7–3.6) of being diagnosed with OAD compared with their unexposed counterparts [13]. By 2016, the prevalence of FDNY physician-diagnosed OAD was 26%, with asthma at 20% as the most common diagnosis (Table 1).

Interstitial Lung Diseases

Interstitial lung diseases (ILD) such as sarcoidosis, pulmonary fibrosis, and bronchiolitis obliterans remain far less common than OAD in our cohort, and, with the exception of sarcoidosis, are extremely rare. In the first 14 years post-9/11, we identified 75 FDNY-WTC responders with new incident sarcoidosis. Pre-9/11, all had normal chest X-rays and normal spirometry and were asymptomatic [14]. This post-9/11 sarcoidosis rate of ~22/100,000 was considerably higher than the average pre-9/11 incidence rate of ~15/100,000. Further, in contrast to pre-9/11 sarcoidosis cases, many FDNY sarcoidosis cases diagnosed post-9/11 were not only symptomatic due primarily to OAD (69%) [14] but also upon further workup, had evidence of cardiac involvement (12%) [15] and/or rheumatologic involvement (15%) [16], the latter often requiring biologicals for disease control.

Upper Respiratory

While not as immediately obvious as a cough and other lower respiratory symptoms, CRS symptoms were also commonly reported by FDNY firefighters and EMS workers. From the first post-9/11 year to 15 years post-9/11, CRS symptoms consistently affected about 40% of the FDNY-WTC rescue/recovery cohort (Fig. 2), in contrast to pre-9/11 reports of frequent rhinosinusitis by 4.4% of FDNY firefighters [17]. Rhinosinusitis symptoms four years post-9/11 were still associated with WTC exposure as measured by both arrival time and duration of work [17].

Examining FDNY medical records, the post-9/11 prevalence of physician-diagnosed CRS increased from 11% in 2005 [18] to 32% in 2016 (Table 1) and was highest in FDNY-WTC responders who arrived either during the morning (36%; Fig. 3) or afternoon of 9/11 (35%). Recent studies confirmed the risk of CRS among early arriving FDNY-WTC responders: firefighters with the earliest arrival time had almost twice the rate of physician-diagnosed CRS when compared with later-arriving firefighters (relative rate: 1.99; 95% CI: 1.64–2.41) [19], and EMS workers with the earliest arrival time had nearly four times the risk of being diagnosed with CRS compared with their unexposed counterparts (relative risk, 3.7; 95% CI, 2.2–6.0) [13].

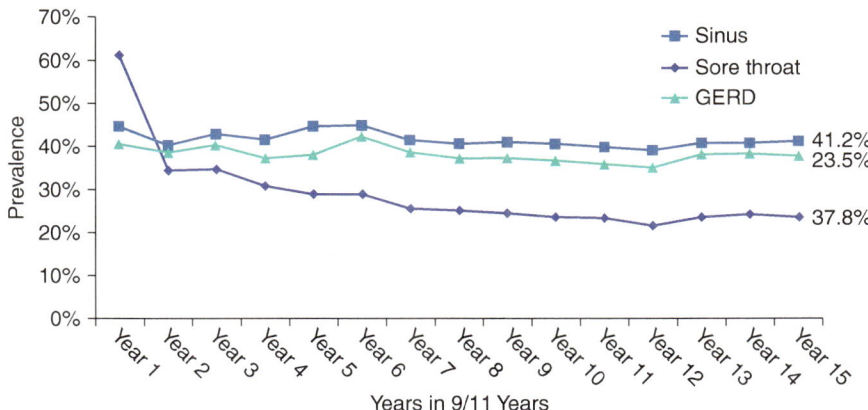

Fig. 2 Prevalence of upper respiratory symptoms by FDNY-WTC responders

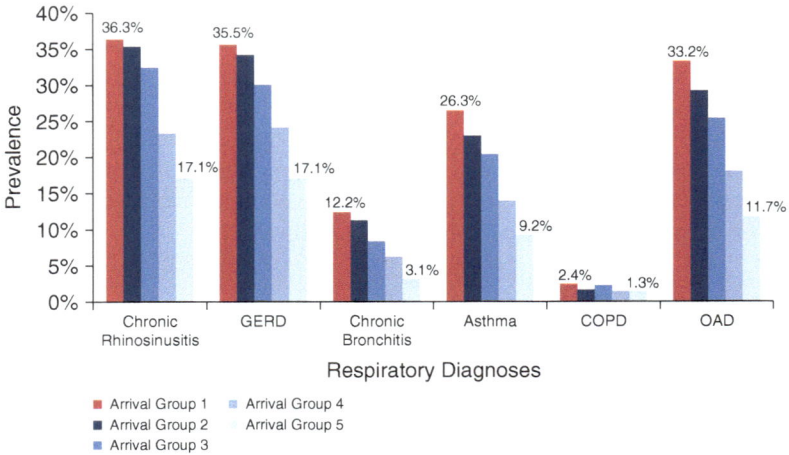

Fig. 3 Post-9/11 prevalence of respiratory health and GERD diagnoses between 2002 and 2015. Note: Arrival Group 1 arrived on the morning of 9/11, Arrival Group 2 arrived during the afternoon of 9/11, Arrival Group 3 arrived on 9/12/2001, Arrival Group 4 arrived any day between 9/13/2001 and 9/24/2001, and Arrival Group 5 arrived after 9/24/2001

GERD

Before 9/11, symptoms consistent with GERD (acid reflux, sore throat, chest burning/tightness, and difficulty swallowing) were reported by 5.2% of FDNY firefighters [17]. However, in the first year post-9/11, 41% reported GERD symptoms, of which sore throat symptoms were the most prevalent (61%; Fig. 2). GERD symptoms, previously shown to be significantly associated with WTC arrival time and duration of work [17], consistently affected about 40% of the FDNY-WTC rescue/recovery cohort (Fig. 2).

The prevalence of FDNY physician-diagnosed GERD was 31% in 2016 (Table 1) and was highest among FDNY-WTC responders with the earliest arrival time (36%; Fig. 3). Firefighters with the earliest arrival time had 1.5 times the rate of having a GERD diagnosis than later-arriving firefighters (relative rate, 1.48; 95% CI, 1.27–1.73) [20], and EMS workers who arrived during the morning of 9/11 had nearly four times the risk of being diagnosed with GERD compared with unexposed EMS (relative risk, 3.8; 95% CI, 2.4–6.1) [13].

Obstructive Sleep Apnea

In 2011, we showed that early arrival time at the WTC site was significantly associated with scoring at high risk for obstructive sleep apnea (OSA) using an adapted Berlin screening survey [21]. In a later study, we confirmed that 81% of 636 participants who scored high risk for OSA had polysomnogram-confirmed OSA [22]. We also found that FDNY responders who arrived at the WTC during the morning of 9/11 had almost twice the odds (OR, 1.91; 95% CI, 1.15–3.17) of polysomnogram-confirmed OSA than those with lower levels of WTC exposure.

Cancer

We showed that seven years after 9/11, FDNY-WTC-exposed firefighters had a 10% higher overall cancer incidence rate (standardized incidence ratio [SIR], 1.10; 95% CI, 0.98–1.25) than the general US male population and a 32% higher rate than in unexposed FDNY firefighters (SIR, 1.32; 95% CI, 1.07–1.62), the latter reaching statistical significance [23]. WTC-exposed firefighters had significantly higher rates for some specific cancers when compared with the general US male population (e.g., prostate [SIR, 1.49; 95% CI, 1.20–1.85] and thyroid [SIR, 3.07; 95% CI, 1.86–5.08]) [23]. In contrast, lung cancer incidence in WTC-exposed firefighters was significantly lower than expected (SIR, 0.42; 95% CI, 0.20–0.86) in the general US male population, likely due to lower smoking rates and the short follow-up period of seven years post-9/11. Two other WTC-exposed cohorts, the WTC Health Consortium and the WTC Health Registry, showed results generally consistent with our findings [4, 5, 24].

Recently, we compared cancer incidence in FDNY-WTC-exposed firefighters to incidence in a combined cohort of career firefighters from Chicago, Philadelphia, and San Francisco [25]. This comparison to firefighters, rather than to the US general population, demonstrated similar, rather than increased, rates of all cancers combined, although rates for thyroid cancer and late-onset prostate cancer remained significantly elevated, similar to our previous results [23].

Autoimmune Diseases

Between 2001 and 2013, we identified 59 FDNY-WTC responders with rheumatologist-confirmed systematic autoimmune disease (SAIDs), of whom 37% had rheumatoid arthritis [26]. In a case-control study, prolonged work at the WTC site was significantly associated with SAIDs: the odds for incident SAIDs increased by 13% (conditional OR, 1.13; 95% CI, 1.02–1.26) for each additional month worked at the site [26].

In a later study, we identified 63 rheumatologist-confirmed cases of SAIDs, but also included 34 additional "probable" cases, that, according to two rheumatologists, likely had SAIDs [27]. Although we found that overall SAIDs rates were not significantly different from expected rates (SIR, 0.97; 95% CI, 0.77–1.21), based on comparison with incident cases from Rochester Epidemiology Project (REP) participants, highly WTC-exposed FDNY responders had an excess of 7.7 cases of SAIDs, while lesser exposed workers had 9.9 fewer cases than expected.

Mental Health

Immediately after 9/11, FDNY-WTC monitoring questionnaires included screening questions for PTSD. In 2005, mental health screening questionnaires were improved and expanded to include validated instruments to assess symptoms consistent with common mental health conditions. The PTSD Checklist (PCL-17) [28] and Center for Epidemiological Studies-Depression scale (CES-D) [29] were used to assess probable PTSD and probable depression, respectively. Before 2005, FDNY assessed probable PTSD using a modified version of the PCL [30]. Alcohol Use Disorders Identification Test (AUDIT) [31] was used to assess harmful alcohol use. Details and scoring of the screening instruments have been previously described [3, 13]. Information from these instruments identified at-risk individuals who were referred to FDNY-CSU. Analyses of these screeners also helped describe the prevalence of probable PTSD, probable depression, and harmful alcohol use and its association with WTC exposure.

Between 2002 and 2005 (years 1 through 4 on Fig. 4), the highest prevalence of probable PTSD was found immediately post-9/11 (10%; Fig. 4) and was especially high among workers with the earliest arrival (25%; data not shown). In fact, this rate of 25% is similar to that reported in survivors of the WTC collapse [32]. In year 15, probable PTSD prevalence was 8% and continued to be higher among workers with the earliest arrival (13%; data not shown). Previous analyses have consistently found an association between PTSD and earliest arrival at the WTC site [13, 30, 33]. Notably, firefighters who arrived during the morning of 9/11 had six times the odds (OR, 6.0; 95% CI, 4.4–8.3) of screening positive for PTSD [33] and EMS workers who arrived during the morning had seven times the risk (OR, 7.0; 95% CI, 3.6–13.5) of screening positive for PTSD [13].

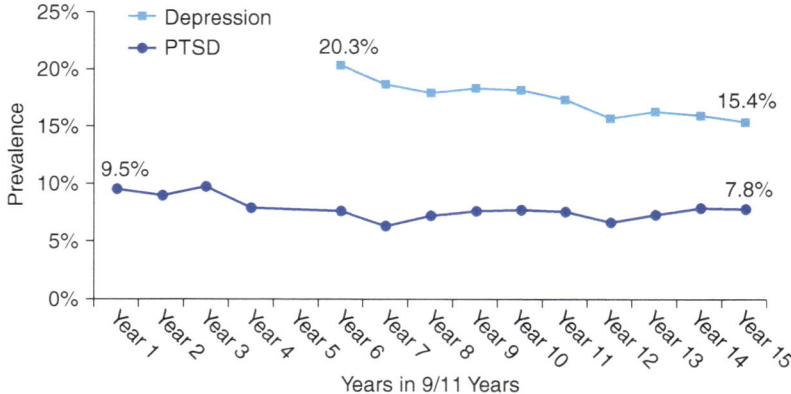

Fig. 4 Probable depression and post-traumatic stress disorder (PTSD) in FDNY-WTC responders. Footnote: PTSD data is unavailable in year 5

High prevalence of probable depression is also documented among FDNY-WTC responders, ranging from 20% in year 6 to 15% in 15 (Fig. 4), and is highest among those with the earliest arrival (20% in year 15; data not shown).

Health Comorbidities

Very substantial comorbidities exist between mental health conditions. Figure 5a shows that, among those who had a mental health questionnaire in year 15, 7% (N = 744) screened positive for both probable PTSD and probable depression. Further, among FDNY-WTC responders with probable PTSD (N = 820), 91% also screened positive for probable depression, and among those with probable depression (N = 1618), 46% also screened positive for probable PTSD. FDNY-WTC responders with harmful alcohol use were twice as likely to screen positive for either PTSD (OR, 2.4; 95% CI, 1.9–4.3) or depression (OR, 1.9; 95% CI, 1.5–2.4) [3].

Physical health conditions also commonly co-occur, such as between WTC cough syndrome and GERD [1] and between CRS, OAD, and GERD [13, 20] (Fig. 5b). By 2016, 1617 (10%) of FDNY-WTC responders had been diagnosed with all three health conditions: CRS, OAD, and GERD (Fig. 5b). Further, 1199 (8%) had both CRS and GERD, 825 (5%) had CRS and OAD, and 692 (4%) had GERD and OAD (Fig. 5b).

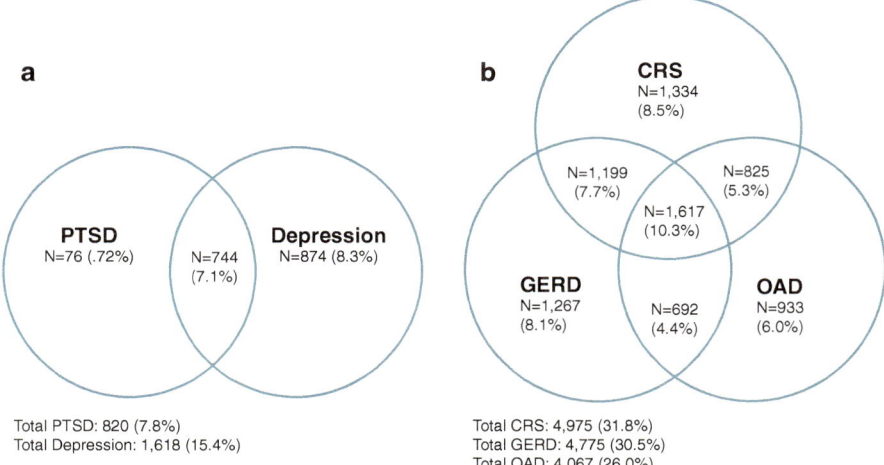

Fig. 5 Mental health (**a**) and physical health (**b**) comorbidities in FDNY-WTC responders. Footnote: Percentages of probable PTSD and probable depression were among N = 10,538 who completed a mental health questionnaire in 9/11 year, year 15 (9/11/2015–9/11/2016). Percentages of CRS, GERD, and OAD were among N = 15,634

Fig. 6 Obstructive airways disease and probable depression comorbidity. Footnote: Percentages were among $N = 15,235$ who ever had a mental health questionnaire

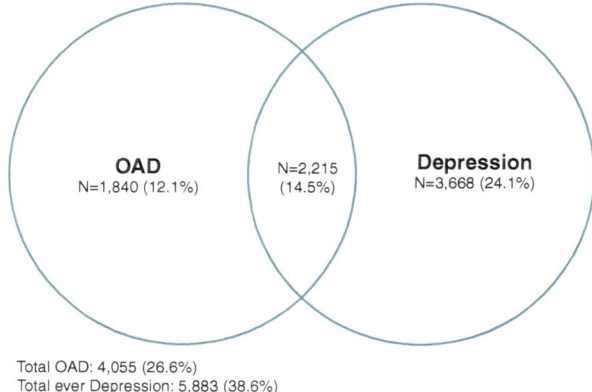

OAD
N=1,840 (12.1%)

N=2,215
(14.5%)

Depression
N=3,668 (24.1%)

Total OAD: 4,055 (26.6%)
Total ever Depression: 5,883 (38.6%)

Importantly, we found that an OAD diagnosis increased the risk of additional diagnoses: firefighters with an OAD diagnosis were more than four times more likely to have a CRS diagnosis (relative rate, 4.15; 95% CI, 3.70–4.66) and more than three times more likely to have a GERD diagnosis (relative rate, 3.18; 95% CI, 2.90–3.48) [20].

Finally, physical and mental health conditions also frequently occur in the same individuals: 15% of those who ever had a mental health questionnaire had both a diagnosis of OAD and reported symptoms consistent with depression (Fig. 6). Nearly 38% of 5883 FDNY-WTC responders who ever screened positive for probable depression also had an OAD diagnosis, and 55% of 4055 workers who had OAD at any time also had probable depression. In another study, we found that firefighters who had probable PTSD shortly after 9/11 had increased odds of WTC cough syndrome up to four years post-9/11 (OR: 1.56; 95% CI: 1.23–1.99) [34]. And among EMS workers who screened positive for PTSD, depression, or harmful alcohol use, 35% had at least one respiratory condition: CRS, GERD, or OAD [13].

Discussion

This report showed that FDNY firefighters and EMS workers with the highest levels of WTC exposure had the greatest risk for adverse health conditions ranging from OAD to PTSD and that, over time, this disproportionate health burden remained. To date, the most highly exposed continue to have the highest prevalence of physician-diagnosed respiratory health conditions such as OAD (33% vs. overall 26%), CRS (36% vs. overall 32%), and GERD (36% vs. overall 31%); 15 years after 9/11, they have the highest prevalence of mental health conditions such as probable PTSD (13% vs. overall 8%) and probable depression (20% vs. overall 15%).

A substantial number of FDNY-WTC responders exhibited impaired pulmonary function. Most of those who experienced an unprecedented decline in lung function shortly after 9/11 continue to show either lack of recovery or only a partial recovery up to 15 years later. Symptoms or diagnoses of respiratory health conditions were rare before 9/11; by 2016, half of the FDNY-WTC rescue/recovery cohort had at least one of the following physician diagnoses: OAD, CRS, or GERD.

The pathophysiological causes of these respiratory conditions, which frequently co-occur in the same individuals, are a topic of intense investigation. Inhalation injuries of toxic, highly alkaline dust at the WTC site, and the lack of personal protective respirators, likely triggered upper and lower respiratory tract injury, inflammation, and symptoms [35]. For the majority of those affected, this has resulted in airways obstruction, as indicated by pulmonary function and methacholine challenge tests and chest CT scans [36]. As for the high incidence of GERD symptoms, ingestion of WTC dust, and other hazardous substances, along with risk factors such as stress in general and PTSD specifically, poor diet, side effects from medications prescribed for WTC-related conditions, and weight gain likely irritated the gastroesophageal tract [1, 35]. Given the observed high comorbidity between GERD, CRS, and OAD, it is unknown whether GERD causes respiratory symptoms or contributes to the persistence of airway inflammation [1, 35]. Nonetheless, WTC treatment guidelines stress that successful management of respiratory conditions is linked to successful treatment of GERD symptoms [35]. It is also important to consider evaluation of possible mental health problems such as PTSD in the treatment of persistent respiratory and GERD conditions, especially given the high comorbidities in this cohort.

Persistence of disease is likely the result of chronic inflammation initiated by exposure to the dust and potentiated by host characteristics as demonstrated by induced sputum studies showing significantly increased percentages of inflammatory biomarkers, neutrophils, and eosinophils in those with high WTC exposure [37] and by serum studies from blood drawn within six months of 9/11 showing elevated levels of known inflammatory biomarkers, such as macrophage-derived chemokines, that were associated with increased risk of subsequent abnormal pulmonary function [38]. The protease/anti-protease imbalance defined by mild to moderate genetic deficiency of alpha-1 antitrypsin deficiency [39] and the elevated set points of eosinophils and IgE levels observed in those with non-resolving upper and lower airways inflammation [40, 41] are intrinsic characteristics of patients that can be assessed repeatedly using inexpensive, commercially available techniques. The ultimate goal of this line of investigation is to develop risk stratification models that allow for more intensive monitoring and treatment of those individuals at the highest risk for WTC-related health effects based not only on WTC-exposure intensity but also on host sensitivity. In so doing, it may also identify targets for more effective therapeutic agents in those with poorly controlled symptoms.

Strengths and Limitations

As described elsewhere [3, 13], our studies may have limitations. First, some of our results may be affected by surveillance bias because the WTCHP schedules periodic monitoring evaluations and provides free treatment for FDNY-WTC responders.

As such, FDNY-WTC responders have increased access to care than the general population. However, we consistently make efforts to address this potential bias. For example, in our cancer studies, we delayed the recorded cancer diagnosis date by two years or more in some analyses and found results similar to those uncorrected for surveillance bias [23, 25].

Another limitation is the lack of a suitable comparison group to WTC-exposed FDNY firefighters. Nearly 99% of the active firefighter workforce participated in the WTC rescue/recovery efforts either on the day of the collapse or in subsequent months. The small minority of firefighters who never worked at the WTC site were older on 9/11 and had worse pre-9/11 health status compared with those who worked at the site, rendering the two groups dissimilar. For that reason, many of our analyses have used external comparison groups including the general US population, REP participants [26], and more recently, NIOSH 3-cities firefighter cohort [25]. Because FDNY-WTC responders had stringent pre-hire health requirements, and were routinely screened post-hire, previous comparisons with the general US male population and REP participants may be limited by dissimilar health status at baseline [3, 27]. The NIOSH 3-cities firefighter cohort, a group more similar to FDNY WTC firefighters, is limited by data that ends in 2009 [25, 42] and an absence of data on smoking status and other potential confounders.

In addition, for mental health conditions, our research studies used validated screening tools rather than physician diagnoses. The use of screeners taken as part of routine monitoring exams, however, may have yielded more in-depth information about the size of the at-risk population. Finally, we acknowledge limited generalizability of our findings to women and minorities and to individuals with lower levels of WTC exposure. The FDNY WTC-exposed cohort is highly exposed and comprised predominantly of white males.

Despite these limitations, FDNY-WTCHP has strengths that enabled us to identify new health conditions and to make causal inferences about the role of WTC exposure in their development. These strengths result from the fact that this cohort existed prior to 9/11, minimizing selection bias, and was served by a pre-existing health infrastructure that had the confidence of both FDNY responders and their leaders to continue serving in this capacity after 9/11. First, because the cohort existed prior to 9/11, we avoided self-selection bias into the FDNY-WTC cohort. Second, because FDNY members had routine health assessments by BHS starting years before 9/11, we have pre-9/11 health information on nearly all of the enrollees, which has allowed us to document the temporal order of disease development in relation to WTC exposure. Third, for physical health conditions, we have direct access to FDNY medical records, which contain FDNY physician diagnoses and clinical data from pulmonary and radiographic tests. Finally, because retirees are included in the program for both monitoring and treatment, the FDNY-WTCHP has minimal longitudinal dropout, thereby allowing health surveillance epidemiologic studies to be more representative of the entire FDNY rescue/recovery cohort.

Conclusion

The collective experience of FDNY-WTCHP physicians and researchers has contributed greatly to the identification and treatment of WTC-related health conditions. FDNY and the FDNY-WTCHP remain committed to providing effective medical care and documenting existing and emergent health conditions for the FDNY-WTC rescue/recovery cohort and, by extension, for all affected individuals in the NYC community and beyond.

Acknowledgments We thank FDNY BHS and World Trade Center Health Programs clinicians for their dedication in providing care for affected FDNY firefighters and EMS workers. We also thank the FDNY data center team and other FDNY researchers for their contributions to data preparation and data analysis. This project was funded by contract # 200-2011-39378 and contract # 200-2011-39383 from the National Institute for Occupational Safety and Health.

References

1. Prezant DJ, Weiden M, Banauch GI, McGuinness G, Rom WN, Aldrich TK, et al. Cough and bronchial responsiveness in firefighters at the World Trade Center site. N Engl J Med. 2002;347(11):806–15.
2. Yip J, Webber MP, Zeig-Owens R, Vossbrinck M, Singh A, Kelly K, et al. FDNY and 9/11: Clinical services and health outcomes in World Trade Center-exposed firefighters and EMS workers from 2001 to 2016. Am J Ind Med. 2016;59(9):695–708.
3. Chiu S, Niles JK, Webber MP, Zeig-Owens R, Gustave J, Lee R, et al. Evaluating risk factors and possible mediation effects in posttraumatic depression and posttraumatic stress disorder comorbidity. Public Health Rep (Washington, DC: 1974). 2011;126(2):201–9.
4. Li J, Cone JE, Kahn AR, Brackbill RM, Farfel MR, Greene CM, et al. Association between World Trade Center exposure and excess cancer risk. JAMA. 2012;308(23):2479–88.
5. Solan S, Wallenstein S, Shapiro M, Teitelbaum SL, Stevenson L, Kochman A, et al. Cancer incidence in world trade center rescue and recovery workers, 2001–2008. Environ Health Perspect. 2013;121(6):699–704.
6. James Zadroga 9/11 Health and Compensation Act of 2010, Pub. L. 111-347, 42 USC §§ 300mm - 300mm-61 (Pub. L. No. 111-347).
7. Aldrich TK, Gustave J, Hall CB, Cohen HW, Webber MP, Zeig-Owens R, et al. Lung function in rescue workers at the World Trade Center after 7 years. N Engl J Med. 2010;362(14):1263–72.
8. Aldrich TK, Vossbrinck M, Zeig-Owens R, Hall CB, Schwartz TM, Moir W, et al. Lung function trajectories in WTC-exposed NYC Firefighters over 13 years: the roles of smoking and smoking cessation. Chest. 2016;149(6):1419–27.
9. Vossbrinck M, Zeig-Owens R, Hall CB, Schwartz T, Moir W, Webber MP, et al. Post-9/11/2001 lung function trajectories by sex and race in World Trade Center-exposed New York City emergency medical service workers. Occup Environ Med. 2016;74(3):200–3.
10. Aldrich TK, Weakley J, Dhar S, Hall CB, Crosse T, Banauch G, et al. Bronchial reactivity and lung function after World Trade Center exposure. Chest. 2016;150(6):1333–40.
11. Banauch GI, Dhala A, Alleyne D, Alva R, Santhyadka G, Krasko A, et al. Bronchial hyper-reactivity and other inhalation lung injuries in rescue/recovery workers after the World Trade Center collapse. Crit Care Med. 2005;33(1 Suppl):S102–6.

12. Glaser MS, Webber MP, Zeig-Owens R, Weakley J, Liu X, Ye F, et al. Estimating the time interval between exposure to the World Trade Center disaster and incident diagnoses of obstructive airway disease. Am J Epidemiol. 2014;180(3):272–9.

13. Yip J, Zeig-Owens R, Webber MP, Kablanian A, Hall CB, Vossbrinck M, et al. World Trade Center-related physical and mental health burden among New York City Fire Department emergency medical service workers. Occup Environ Med. 2015;73(1):13–20.

14. Izbicki G, Chavko R, Banauch GI, Weiden MD, Berger KI, Aldrich TK, et al. World Trade Center "sarcoid-like" granulomatous pulmonary disease in New York City Fire Department rescue workers. Chest. 2007;131(5):1414–23.

15. Hena K, Yip J, Jaber N, et al. Clinical characteristics of sarcoidosis in World Trade Center (WTC) exposed Fire Department of the City of New York (FDNY) firefighters. Chest. 2016;150(4):514A.

16. Loupasakis K, Berman J, Jaber N, Zeig-Owens R, Webber MP, Glaser MS, et al. Refractory sarcoid arthritis in World Trade Center-exposed New York City firefighters: a case series. J Clin Rheumatol Pract Rep Rheum Musculoskelet Dis. 2015;21(1):19–23.

17. Webber MP, Gustave J, Lee R, Niles JK, Kelly K, Cohen HW, et al. Trends in respiratory symptoms of firefighters exposed to the world trade center disaster: 2001–2005. Environ Health Perspect. 2009;117(6):975–80.

18. Niles JK, Webber MP, Liu X, Zeig-Owens R, Hall CB, Cohen HW, et al. The upper respiratory pyramid: early factors and later treatment utilization in World Trade Center exposed firefighters. Am J Ind Med. 2014;57(8):857–65.

19. Weakley J, Hall CB, Liu X, Zeig-Owens R, Webber MP, Schwartz T, et al. The effect of World Trade Center exposure on the latency of chronic rhinosinusitis diagnoses in New York City firefighters: 2001–2011. Occup Environ Med. 2016;73(4):280–3.

20. Liu X, Zeig-Owens R, Weakley J, Webber MP, Schwartz TM, Prezant DJ, et al., editors. The effect of World Trade Center exposure on the timing of aerodigestive diagnoses in New York City Firefighters: 2001–2011. New York, NY: New York City Epidemiology Forum; 2016.

21. Webber MP, Lee R, Soo J, Gustave J, Hall CB, Kelly K, et al. Prevalence and incidence of high risk for obstructive sleep apnea in World Trade Center-exposed rescue/recovery workers. Sleep Breathing = Schlaf Atmung. 2011;15(3):283–94.

22. Glaser MS, Shah N, Webber MP, Zeig-Owens R, Jaber N, Appel DW, et al. Obstructive sleep apnea and World Trade Center exposure. J Occup Environ Med/Am Coll Occup Environ Med. 2014;56(Suppl 10):S30–4.

23. Zeig-Owens R, Webber MP, Hall CB, Schwartz T, Jaber N, Weakley J, et al. Early assessment of cancer outcomes in New York City firefighters after the 9/11 attacks: an observational cohort study. Lancet. 2011;378(9794):898–905.

24. Boffetta P, Zeig-Owens R, Wallenstein S, Li J, Brackbill R, Cone J, et al. Cancer in World Trade Center responders: findings from multiple cohorts and options for future study. Am J Ind Med. 2016;59(2):96–105.

25. Moir W, Zeig-Owens R, Daniels RD, Hall CB, Webber MP, Jaber N, et al. Post-9/11 cancer incidence in World Trade Center-exposed New York City firefighters as compared to a pooled cohort of firefighters from San Francisco, Chicago and Philadelphia (9/11/2001–2009). Am J Ind Med. 2016;59(9):722–30.

26. Webber MP, Moir W, Zeig-Owens R, Glaser MS, Jaber N, Hall C, et al. Nested case-control study of selected systemic autoimmune diseases in World Trade Center rescue/recovery workers. Arthritis Rheumatol (Hoboken, NJ). 2015;67(5):1369–76.

27. Webber MP, Moir W, Crowson CS, Cohen HW, Zeig-Owens R, Hall CB, et al. Post-September 11, 2001, incidence of systemic autoimmune diseases in World Trade Center-exposed firefighters and emergency medical service workers. Mayo Clin Proc. 2016;91(1):23–32.

28. Weathers F, Litz B, Herman D, Huska J, Keane T, editors. The PTSD checklist (PCL): reliability, validity, and diagnostic utility. In: Annual meeting of the international society of traumatic stress studies, San Francisco, TX, 1993.

29. Radloff LS. The CES-D scale a self-report depression scale for research in the general population. Appl Psycholog Meas. 1977;1(3):385–401.

30. Soo J, Webber MP, Gustave J, Lee R, Hall CB, Cohen HW, et al. Trends in probable PTSD in firefighters exposed to the World Trade Center disaster, 2001–2010. Disaster Med Public Health Prep. 2011;5(Suppl 2):S197–203.
31. Babor TF, Higgins-Biddle JC, Saunders JB, Monteiro MG. The alcohol use disorders identification test: guidelines for use in primary care, 2nd ed. Geneva: World Health Organization; 2001.
32. Brackbill RM, Cone JE, Farfel MR, Stellman SD. Chronic physical health consequences of being injured during the terrorist attacks on World Trade Center on September 11, 2001. Am J Epidemiol. 2014;179(9):1076–85.
33. Berninger A, Webber MP, Cohen HW, Gustave J, Lee R, Niles JK, et al. Trends of elevated PTSD risk in firefighters exposed to the World Trade Center disaster: 2001–2005. Public Health Rep. 2010;125(4):556–66.
34. Niles JK, Webber MP, Gustave J, Cohen HW, Zeig-Owens R, Kelly KJ, et al. Comorbid trends in World Trade Center cough syndrome and probable posttraumatic stress disorder in firefighters. Chest. 2011;140(5):1146–54.
35. Prezant DJ, Levin S, Kelly KJ, Aldrich TK. Upper and lower respiratory diseases after occupational and environmental disasters. Mt Sinai J Med NY. 2008;75(2):89–100.
36. Weiden MD, Ferrier N, Nolan A, Rom WN, Comfort A, Gustave J, et al. Obstructive airways disease with air trapping among firefighters exposed to World Trade Center dust. Chest. 2010;137(3):566–74.
37. Fireman EM, Lerman Y, Ganor E, Greif J, Fireman-Shoresh S, Lioy PJ, et al. Induced sputum assessment in New York City firefighters exposed to World Trade Center dust. Environ Health Perspect. 2004;112(15):1564–9.
38. Nolan A, Naveed B, Comfort AL, Ferrier N, Hall CB, Kwon S, et al. Inflammatory biomarkers predict airflow obstruction after exposure to World Trade Center dust. Chest. 2012;142(2):412–8.
39. Banauch GI, Brantly M, Izbicki G, Hall C, Shanske A, Chavko R, et al. Accelerated spirometric decline in New York City firefighters with alpha(1)-antitrypsin deficiency. Chest. 2010;138(5):1116–24.
40. Kazeros A, Maa MT, Patrawalla P, Liu M, Shao Y, Qian M, et al. Elevated peripheral eosinophils are associated with new-onset and persistent wheeze and airflow obstruction in world trade center-exposed individuals. J Asthma Off J Assoc Care of Asthma. 2013;50(1):25–32.
41. Kwon S, Putman B, Weakley J, Hall CB, Zeig-Owens R, Schwartz T, et al. Blood eosinophils and World Trade Center exposure predict surgery in chronic rhinosinusitis: a 13.5-year longitudinal study. Ann Am Thorac Soc. 2016;13(8):1253–61.
42. Daniels RD, Kubale TL, Yiin JH, Dahm MM, Hales TR, Baris D, et al. Mortality and cancer incidence in a pooled cohort of US firefighters from San Francisco, Chicago and Philadelphia (1950–2009). Occup Environ Med. 2014;71(6):388–97.

Index